Reflective Leadership in Healthcare

This practical and positive guide shows how good, effective reflection can help people to stay on track, as well as understand what is working well and what might be improved – essential skills for leaders at all levels of practice from newly qualified staff to senior managers.

Supporting readers to link theory and action with reflection, the authors illustrate how practitioners can exercise their own kinds of leadership to strengthen, improve and thrive. Taking a realistic and achievable view of leadership, the book:

- reviews the different leadership approaches and styles that help to inform us about what makes a good leader;
- explores the role of emotional intelligence, appreciative intelligence and narrative intelligence in leadership, especially in complex, challenging and continually changing healthcare settings; and
- uses case studies and practice examples to ensure the book is relevant, current and helpful.

Reflective leadership is fundamental to providing safe, effective healthcare to all patients, as well as enhancing resilience for individuals, teams and organisations. This guide is an essential read for healthcare students and practitioners, no matter at what stage or level they are at as a leader.

Rhian Last is a Nurse Educator, currently General Practice Nurse Facilitator at Leeds Community Healthcare NHS Trust and a RCGP Yorkshire Faculty Board Member.

Sue Lillyman is an Associate Lecturer at both the University of Worcester, UK and Education for Health.

Reflective Leadership in Healthcare

A Practical Guide

Rhian Last and Sue Lillyman

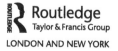
Routledge
Taylor & Francis Group

LONDON AND NEW YORK

Cover image: © Getty Images

First published 2024
by Routledge
4 Park Square, Milton Park, Abingdon, Oxon OX14 4RN

and by Routledge
605 Third Avenue, New York, NY 10158

Routledge is an imprint of the Taylor & Francis Group, an informa business

British Library Cataloguing-in-Publication Data
A catalogue record for this book is available from the British Library

Library of Congress Cataloging-in-Publication Data
Names: Last, Rhian, author. | Lillyman, Sue, author.
Title: Reflective leadership in healthcare : a practical guide /
Rhian Last, Sue Lillyman.
Description: Abingdon, Oxon ; New York, NY : Routledge, 2024. |
Includes bibliographical references and index.
Identifiers: LCCN 2023007634 | ISBN 9781032349398 (hardback) |
ISBN 9781032349367 (paperback) | ISBN 9781003324560 (ebook)
Subjects: LCSH: Health services administration. |
Hospitals--Administration. | Leadership.
Classification: LCC RA971 .L323 2024 |
DDC 362.1068--dc23/eng/20230527
LC record available at https://lccn.loc.gov/2023007634

ISBN: 978-1-032-34939-8 (hbk)
ISBN: 978-1-032-34936-7 (pbk)
ISBN: 978-1-003-32456-0 (ebk)

DOI: 10.4324/9781003324560

Typeset in Helvetica
by MPS Limited, Dehradun

Contents

Preface

Although we may not all aspire to be the leader of big organisations we can all be leaders in different aspects of our lives. This may be within a social group where we may have responsibilities for example leading a club, organising events or mobilising teams or it may be work-based where we lead a team through a specific project, in everyday practice or in a leadership role. It may, or may not, be part of our role description but we are all part of the change that goes on in our lives. As we know all organisations experience change, whatever size, and if we work in them then we are also part of that change process. We may be the leader or a follower in the process of change, whichever role we take we need to understand what is happening and be engaged in the process as Goleman (2000) reminds us it is how we do it that will result in our success.

This book reviews the different leadership approaches and styles that help to inform us about what makes a good leader. It will help people on their journey no matter at what stage or level they are at as a leader.

Most of what we know about leadership and management, according to Ellis and Abbott (2013), is based on theory, supposition and experience. Through this book, we will bring these three aspects together to build on them and identify ways forward for all members, at all levels, of any organisation to function as effective leaders within their roles.

Chapter 1
New thinking about leaders and leadership

Being a leader is not just for the good and great of the country or organisation, we are all leaders at some time in our lives either at home or in the workplace. As stated in the introduction, in your social life it may be as part of leading a discussion, a social group/sports event, volunteer organisation, project, etc. or within the workplace, it maybe as part of leading a specific project or a small group of people in everyday work. It could also be part of your job description when you have a specific leadership role in relation to work areas, group of people or the whole organisation. Whatever reason we take on the leadership role Northouse (2012) reminds us that it is challenging, exciting, rewarding and with it there are many responsibilities.

To begin with we identify what leadership is and what we mean by being a leader. At this point, we also need to differentiate between leadership and management.

Leadership

Leadership is a contested notion (Southworth 1998; Kings Fund 2011) and often conceived as a function rather than a role (Warwick and Swaffield 2006). It originated in the eighteenth century (Patel et al 2010) and has changed in its approach over the centuries. However, it was during the twentieth century, with the development of social science, that leadership became more prolific and emerged within every discipline according to Northouse (2012). During this long history, there have also been many changes in its approach resulting in

DOI: 10.4324/9781003324560-1

different definitions of the term. Bass (1981) stated that there are as many different definitions as there are persons who have attempted to define it. However, most authors agree that leadership is an act or process of working with and influencing others towards a shared goal (Stogdill 1950; Hemphill and Coons 1957; Hollander 1978; Rauch and Behling 1984; Hersey and Blanchard 1988; Cohen 1990; Kouzes and Posner 1995; Ellis and Abbot 2013).

At this juncture it is important to note that leadership should not be confused with management. Managers have the authority to get others to do things for them and have the power to enforce change (Ellis and Abbot 2013). The manager therefore is usually concerned with operational issues holding positions of seniority. However, leadership is not related to a position of power or authority but more about working with others towards a shared goal. Although leadership and management can be two different roles/ people both terms are used interchangeably and as Ellis and Abbot (2013) note best managers are also good leaders.

Purpose of leadership

Although, as stated above, there are many definitions authors often agree that it involves leaders and followers, intends real change, involves social order, situates within specific local and idiosyncratic context, provides direction and involves relationships between individuals with how they engage and behave together (Cardoso et al 2013; Edmonstone 2013; Patel et al 2010; Ellis and Abbot 2013).

Leaders

Leaders then are the people/person that takes that change forward. John Kotter stated in his definition that a leader envisions the future and situates others with this vision, inspiring and motivating them to overcome challenges (Kotter 2012). Northouse (2012) also provides a summary of the leader stating that they have the ability, skills, behaviour, relationships and influencing processes.

Knowing what leadership is and what a leader is there are many different styles of leadership and traits of a leader. Northouse (2012) stated that these traits are the distinguishing qualities of the leader. In the next section, we are going to look at some of the leadership styles that can be seen in some of our leaders and managers.

Leadership styles

We have all seen, and worked for, great leaders and also those who have not been so successful in their role. The complexities of leadership are often due to the interconnections between power, authority, the system and emotion and how it is all transmitted (Nicholson et al 2011). As Blanken (2019) reminds us, there is a time and place for all types of leaders and none of them is good or bad, but it is how leaders use the different approaches that determine the outcome.

Many organisations are complex and need to be run with high-quality management and leadership and therefore the leaders need to generate their own leadership style (Stelter and Law 2010). However new leadership approaches also need to embrace the different leadership behaviours and create a supportive leadership community which includes compassion, respect and humanity from all levels within the system, including those who are on the front line (Storey and Holti 2013). Therefore, it is important to review all the styles, characteristics and traits of a leader, not because of the differences over time, but because a good leader will adapt and utilise different styles and behaviours for particular situations.

Below we have reviewed the literature to identify the different styles; however, Warwick and Swaffield (2006) remind us that often these lists are produced without considering the context. We therefore recognise that these definitions are outside of any context and that there is no single style that suits all situations within the complex organisations in which we work. We also need to remember that no one style can consistently produce better results than another and even the research findings remain inconsistent in their effectiveness of the different styles (Blanken 2019; Gill 2011). However, as Currie et al (2009) and Schilling (2009) found, whichever leadership approach is used there is a direct effect on the organisations performance whether that is for good or ill and the goals of that organisation should be at the heart of the relationship between the effective leader and the follower.

The most common types of leadership approaches listed in the literature include:

- Autocratic

Also referred to as authoritarian (position based) leadership (Gill 2011).

This approach to leadership is seen where the leader makes the decisions on their own without any input from others and where the leaders tend to control their staff by giving directions, setting goals and structuring their work (Northouse 2014). It is a rule-focused approach to leadership with a top-down flow of command and communication where the leader exercises ultimate power in decision making (Barr and Dowding 2012). However, this type of approach is often used effectively in a situation of real urgency where there is no time for discussion or when safety may be compromised (Blanken 2019). When used continuously, Leech (2012) points out that, this can lead to a 'responsibility vacuum' where there is a danger of not using common sense decisions that may be put forward by the staff. This he argues may result in a 'them and us' culture that breeds rumour and speculation.

- Laissez-Faire

This style, according to Gill (2011), is non-transactional although he questions if it is a leadership style at all. However, the leader conscientiously passes the decision-making process to their subordinates in a genuine laissez-faire style, according to Barr and Dowding (2012), as opposed to being a non-leader who does not engage in the decision-making process. Although this leader knows what is happening and will monitor performance by giving feedback regularly (Blanken 2019) they do not nurture or guide their staff and have minimal influence and engagement (Northouse

2014), giving their employees ultimate freedom (Jones and Bennett 2012). Blanken (2019) suggests this style is often useful when there is an effective, experienced skilled team and where the autonomy of team leaders can lead to high job satisfaction and where there is a highly skilled and experienced staff who have a drive to work effectively. However, it is less effective when staff feel insecure at the unavailability of, or access to, the manager.

• Transactional

This approach is based on the work of Bass (1985) from his work in the 1960s and 1980s at a time when there was more stability in employment (Barr and Dowding 2012). In this approach, the leader provides material, or psychological rewards, and/or punishments in return for compliance of the staff (Gill 2011; Jones and Bennett 2012). Self-predetermined goals are set together with the workers in order to get things done to meet the organisational goals with a more task orientated, following the rules, approach (Barr and Dowding 2012). This has been seen more in modern healthcare with the introduction of targets that are set and penalties that are incurred for non-achievement (Jones and Bennett 2012).

• Democratic

This approach, often called participative, is where the leader values the input of others and shares responsibility, consultation and delegation and provides feedback (Jones and Bennett 2012). They work with their staff but treat them as being fully capable of carrying out work on their own (Northouse 2014). It is where consensus is sought with commitment through ownership and teamwork (Barr and Dowding 2012). Staff are encouraged to be part of the decision-making process and in turn are kept informed about anything that affects their work and encourages them in that. It can also be effective with complex problems that require more input. It can lead to more job satisfaction and encourages team building. However, it is less effective when there are time constraints and where mistakes cannot be made, especially where staff safety is a critical concern.

- Transformational   This approach to leadership was first coined by Downtown in 1973 and was highlighted by Burns in 1978. These leaders raise people's motivation and promote a higher sense of purpose (Gill 2011) and are concerned with engaging the hearts and minds of their staff (Jones and Bennett 2012). There is a high level of communication from management to meet goals and the leader motivates the employees through communication and high visibility. They engage in active listening, identify personal concerns, needs and abilities of their staff whilst their aim is to develop their staff (Gill 2011). In this approach, the teams are more diffuse and there is a distributed model of leadership that is operated within an organisational context (Nicholson et al 2011). Bamford-Wade and Moss (2010) used four i's to identify the transformative leader and include: idealised influence, inspirational motivation, intellectual stimulation and individual consideration.

Having reviewed the more common styles of leadership above we have included some of the newer paradigms that can be seen in practice today below including:

- Servant   This approach was first coined by Greenleaf in 1970 where the leader places the needs of the staff first and is based on a humanistic approach (Greenleaf 1991). These leaders see themselves as stewards of resources including human, financial or otherwise

(Chen et al 2013). The approach is one of being; one who serves first with service at the core according to Chen et al (2013) and Mahon (2011) and with, what Waterman (2011) refers to as, having a 'servant heart'. This leader also develops a mutually empowering relationship where they are able to articulate the vision and goals that are based on the values their followers trust (Gresh 2006). The servant leader acts socially rather than selfishly and is orientated towards moral authority with an emphasis towards positive values such as trust, honesty and fairness (Chen et al 2013). They care deeply about people and create an environment where people can fulfil their potential (Thornton 2013) and, in doing so, place the needs of their followers first by inspiring their subordinates to generate better awareness, trust, learning and spiritual fulfilment at work (Chen et al 2013). They do this whilst also enhancing professionalism (Gresh 2006) and producing and enabling change rather than adopting a hierarchical approach (Waterman 2011). This leader is creative, visionary and often has foresight, followers often regard them with trust, belief and there is a sense of being part of a team (Waterman 2011). They come from a horizontally orientated leadership position where colleagues are helped to become the best they can be (Mahon 2011). Ultimately the servant leader serves and supports teams and works for the common good (Jones 2008).

- Level 5 leadership
This was introduced by Jim Collins (2001) in his book 'Good to be great'. It consists of five levels of leadership in the form of a hierarchy of executive capabilities with level 5 at the top. These level 5 leaders, according to Greenstein (2012), embody the paradoxical mix of professional will and personal humanity. They attend to people first and strategy second (Thomas 2005). They nurture their staff and do not seek credit but aim to develop an organisation that runs well after they have gone (Caulkins 2008,

Greenstein 2012). They demonstrate characteristics of low charisma and high determination (Caulkins 2008) and through their desire to lead they build the company that thinks from a place of opportunity, in doing so they are not afraid to hire people with more qualifications than themselves or are more experienced in order to meet the organisations goals (Greenstein 2012).

- Situational This approach is where the leader adjusts their leadership style to the situation and links behaviours with the groups readiness, is supporting, while empowering and includes coaching (Blanken 2019). It enables leaders to identify tasks whilst determining the groups maturity, selecting appropriate styles and modifying them according to the situation (Waller et al 1989).

Other approaches you may come across in the literature also include:

- Paternalistic Where the leader is acting as the parent with concern for their staff and includes the paternalism and decision making on behalf of other people (Barr and Dowding 2012).
- Quantum This is based on quantum thinking, a belief that everything relates each other with a focus on life's continuum but is non-linear (Porter-O'Grady and Malloch 2016). The future is anticipated and value-driven actions are addressed. This is viewed as a multifocal process that includes multisystem within systems. The leader thinks ahead and forms different scenarios of what might happen. They encourage questioning, experiments and thrive on uncertainty with a willingness to learn and changing dependency from past practice (Watson et al 2018).
- Compassionate This approach rejects the heroic model of leadership and is based on a shared, distributed and adaptive approach. It involves the creation of

systems that harness positive adaptive responses to change whilst containing anxiety and supporting the individual (de Zulueta 2016). With quality of care at the heart of this approach the aim is to empower people to deliver care together through trust, understanding, the building of inclusions and reduction of inequalities (NHS England 2023).

- Toxic

The approach is associated with bullying, toxic ambivalence, authoritative, abusive and demeaning approach to their staff and organisations (Johnson 2012). Toxic leaders are often disinterested in individuals' development and can be impulsive and unpredictable with little awareness of their impact on others (Wasylyshyn et al 2012).

- Distributive

Also called 'dispersed', 'collective' or 'supportive' (Elmore 2004) where there is a sharing of leadership between individuals who jointly generate commitment, cohesion and wisdom (Grint 2005; Bennett et al 2003) giving followers active roles, ownership and a voice in decision making (McCombe 2013). This approach, according to Jones (2008), focuses on the fluidity, sharing roles, harnessing expertise, opening up boundaries and collegiality.

- Primal leadership

This style of leadership was first coined by Goleman et al (2002) in their model of leadership where emotional intelligence is applied to leadership.

- Strategic

This includes many definitions according to Gill (2011) and is usually used in large corporations and the military. It stresses a competitive nature and is concerned with developing the organisations vision, mission, strategy and cultures. Decision making is seen as a key competence in the strategic leader (Gill 2011).

- Team

  This is where supervisors have been replaced with the team approach to leadership and where there is a notion of distribution leadership (Barr and Dowding 2012). This approach involves giving power to everyone and that can be at different levels such as; executive teams, district teams or local/community teams. Those who work in teams have also reported a higher level of commitment to their work with lower stress levels (Davies 2013). Davies also found that this was the best way to implement strategies as it provides consistency within the organisation.

- Coaching

  This approach involves the ability to train and teach. It includes narrative collaborative practice which can support self-created and reflective leaders (Stelter and Law 2010).

- Dialogical

  This includes a more appreciative interaction with listening and equal participation for all the groups (Yliruka and Karvinen-Niikoski 2013). It encourages the whole workforce to utilise their expertise.

- Eco leadership

  With the increasing awareness of sustainability, this approach focuses on the ecosystem within wider ecosystems and the connectivity and interdependence of these. It is an integrated approach that is centred around sustainability but includes values, collaboration, justice, advocacy and, when and if needed activism, (McKimm and McLean 2020).

- Multi-dimensional

  Used in teams where there are different disciplines and skill mix. It is seen in clinical leadership within the NHS. It is achieved through emotional intelligence and involves a leader who is caring, compassionate and can effectively and confidently transform community services (Leigh et al 2014).

These approaches are not seen in their pure sense but often overlap and have been further categorised into four types of leaders, as opposed to approaches to leadership by Thornton (2013) as:

- Thought leaders
- Courageous leaders
- Inspirational leaders
- Servant leaders

For Thornton, the 'thought leaders' are those who actualise change through stretching their followers to envision new possibilities. 'Courageous leaders', he identifies, as those who go ahead in the face of considerable opposition and risk. The 'inspirational leader' is the one who promotes change through the passion of their own commitment to ideas and ideals whilst the 'servant leaders' care about the people they work with and strive to remove any barriers and obstacles that may hold their followers back from achieving their full potential.

Other authors, such as Gill (2011), use categories of:

- Visionary leadership
- Charismatic leaders
- Organic leadership
- Centred leadership
- Pragmatic leadership
- Warrior leadership
- Strategic leadership
- Evolutionary

These, Gill (2011) notes, are associated with the transformational leader where leadership behaviours are centred on empowerment, motivation and inspiration.

As stated above and as Thornton (2013) noted, many leaders use a combination of two or more leadership types. We also note that there is a time and place for all types of leaders and it is how we use the approach to the leadership role that determines our success, or failure, as a leader.

Traits of the leader

Other authors also offer us lists of characteristics, traits or qualities for a good leader which include:

- Empathy
- Consistency
- Honesty
- Direction
- Communication
- Flexibility
- Conviction
- Ability to delegate
- Sense of humour
- Confidence
- Commitment
- Positive attitude
- Creativity
- Intuition
- Ability to inspire

The list goes on …

In this book, we will draw on some of the approaches, types, characteristics, traits and qualities mentioned above that enhance a positive, supportive and strengths-based leader. As leaders, we can make a difference in practice, as well as inspire and support others working within a specific environment, whilst also meeting the new approach to leadership within our organisation.

Changing leadership approaches within healthcare

In order to see how these leadership styles can be changed and/or be influenced by polices, reviews and time, we have included, as an exemplar, an overview of the NHS since its inception in 1948.

In a system such as the National Health Service, from its inception in 1948 when it was based on a liberal socialist ideology of health that was the right for all people regardless of their ability to pay, it has changed to what today is often seen by the public as almost a religion or system of belief (Barr and Dowding 2012). Through these changes, we have witnessed various approaches to leadership. By reviewing how, and why, these leadership approaches have changed we can begin to understand where the service has come from and, by understanding these changes, we can highlight the different traits and characteristics of the managers and leaders that have helped form the NHS of today.

In the NHS of 1948, the leadership style of the day was that of an autocratic 'great-man' trait with a 'hard-nosed' scientific approach to leadership that often reviewed the organisation as a machine (Nicholson et al 2011). However, since then we have seen changes in the service management and leadership styles, influenced through several key reports and reforms, which have had a profound effect on how the leadership approach has changed and adapted over the years.

These major reports date back to the Porritt Report in 1962. At this time, the British Medical Association Committee Inquiry into the NHS suggested services should be brought together under a single area board which would be a representation of the professions with a doctor as the Chief Officer (Porritt 1962). Then in 1966, the Salmon report was introduced which aimed at raising the profile of nursing, especially in hospital management, with the introduction of a Chief Nursing Officer (Ministry of Health and Scottish Home and Health Departments 1966). A year later the Cogwheel Report called for even more clinicians to be involved in management (Ministry of Health 1967) and the King's Fund/Institute of Hospital Administrators Joint Working Party wanted a clear chain of command and introduced a general manager who would be supported by medical and nursing directors with additional support from a director of finance, statistical services and a director of general services (Howard 1967). Although this resulted in a more distributed approach to leadership at the time, with a shared leadership approach, the 'situational leadership approach' was also more evident where the leaders adapted their leadership style to the situation at hand (Grint 2005).

In 1972, the 'Grey Book' recommended a more multidisciplinary approach that would include an administrator, treasurer, nurse and doctors (DHSS 1972) and 1973 saw the NHS Reorganisation Act

(1973) which created 14 Regional Health Authorities and 90 Area Health Authorities, each with a Chair and non-executive members, devolving the leadership role further down the service line. However, in 1979, the Royal Commission rejected general (as opposed to consensus) management in the NHS and in 1980, the Health Services Act created 192 District Health Authorities in England which devolved management down into even smaller units. By 1983, the Griffiths Report found that the NHS had no coherent system of management and recommended that general managers be introduced into the NHS. In the early 1990s, there was another shift in the leadership approach to healthcare as the Working for Patients (DoH 1989) and the NHS and Community Care Act (DoH 1990) proposed the introduction of an internal market which separated the purchasers from providers of services and GPs were given the option of becoming fund holders (Department of Health 1989). As well as this GP-led management it was mandatory for hospitals to have medical directors on their boards (Moll et al 2011) and by 1994 practice-based commissioning was introduced. At this time, the regional health authorities were abolished with eight regional offices being created and there was a merger of the district health authorities and family health services (Managing the New NHS 1993 and the Health Authorities Act 1995, Department of Health 1993). By the end of the 1990s, the Health Act (1999) introduced the National Institute for Clinical Excellence and established the Commission for Health Improvement (later the Healthcare Commission) at the same time removing the GP fundholding within primary care groups.

For the new millennium, the NHS Plan (DoH 2000) introduced performance targets and standards with an annual assessment of NHS organisations. This was reviewed in 2008 in the Darzi report, NHS Next Stage Review (DoH 2008) which placed a greater emphasis on clinical leadership and highlighted the importance of effective leadership including a greater involvement of clinicians (Nicholson et al 2011). The National Leadership Council was also established by the NHS's Chief Executive along with the NHS Leadership Qualities Framework (DoH and National Skills Academy for Social Care 2004) which was built on the medical competence framework. This framework included leadership competencies that were incorporated into the training and education of all clinical professionals and emphasised situational leadership (Nicholson et al 2011). Sherring (2012) argues that it was through the NHS guidance in 2009 they began to understand the importance of leadership. David Nicholson in 2009, the then CEO of the NHS, built on Darzi's report through Inspiring Leaders: Leadership for Quality (DoH 2009) which charged the Strategic Health Authorities to fill the gaps in leadership as well as to nurture potential talent across the NHS.

In 2010, the government set out more radical plans to reform the NHS through their Health and Social Care Bill, Liberating the NHS (DoH 2010) by shifting the power of accountability and by removing the Strategic Health Authorities and Primary Care Trusts and replacing them with the National Commissions Board and introducing local consortia of GPs that would carry out the commissioning of services. Trusts could also seek foundation status which would then be a regulated market in the provision of healthcare and saw the introduction of mutual and social enterprises being introduced into the healthcare system.

The Kings Fund (2011), in their report, also noted that it is essential that there was a clear national focus for leadership and development to take the NHS forward in the twenty-first century with a shift towards autonomy, responsibility and accountability towards patient care and compassion (Storey and Holti 2013). This also includes what Barr and Dowding (2012) refer to as a 'growth culture' where emotional intelligence is developed and incorporated into the leadership approach. However, safety was to remain at the heart and a central theme of leadership (Kings Fund 2011; Francis Report 2013) and we must continue to learn from the past.

Following a review of the leadership needs of the NHS in 2011 the Kings Fund reported on their findings and highlighted that the leadership style needed to change from the 'hero' approach, when they suggest that serious misjudgements can be made, to a more 'board to ward' approach where every provider and clinician takes responsibility for the leadership and management delivery. This approach is based on shared leadership with a focus on developing teams and individuals across the systems of care which includes 'followership' as well as leadership (Kings Fund 2011). This approach of back to the floor has also been seen in a number of industries (Stagecoach Group 2012) and, according to Sofarelli and

Brown (1998), refers to a leadership-focused health service system where Michie and West (2004) and Carroll et al (2008) stated that the culture, climate and structure has an impact on the people who work within it. In 2013, the Berwick Report also recommended the move from the board room to the bedside in an attempt to address safety and clearly outlined leadership at every level. In this journey to putting patients first, endorsed by the DoH (2013), there was an attempt to make the organisation transparent with a learning culture and accountability that was taken from the patient's perspectives. The Keogh review (2013) also led to some of these changes due to the high mortality rate that they found in 14 NHS and foundation trusts.

Alongside in 2013, the NHS Leadership Academy produced a further healthcare leadership model for all the members in which they included the nine dimensions of; confidence and show empathy, be punctual and show forgiveness, be proud and show humility, be disciplined and show humanity, be recognised and show recognition, be bold and show discretion, be spontaneous and show thoughtfulness, be directed and show consideration, be firm and show compassion, be generous and show gratitude, be a listener and show appreciation and be a leader and show compliance. They also emphasised the need for self-awareness, self-confidence, self-control, self-knowledge, personal reflection, resilience and determination (NHS Leadership Academy 2013a, 2013b). There was also the introduction of a new fast-track leadership development scheme for NHS England which aimed to combine the development of senior NHS clinicians with those outside the NHS (Edmonstone 2013). In this process, the participants were promoted rapidly into senior managers and chief executive roles (Lintern 2013); this was also based on the acquisition of academic qualifications (Edmonstone 2013). However, Edmonstone (2013) argues that there is no guarantee that through the enhancement of the individual-based approach to developing leaders develops relationship-based social capital.

All the changes noted recently have been made in the wake of the Francis report when there was a move to adopt a culture of safety, learning and transparency within the NHS (Muls et al 2015). In 2015, the Duty of Candour (Care Quality Commission 2015) was also viewed as a mechanism to support this cultural change and assist with the bottom-up approach to leadership and the continual improvement process (Muls et al 2015).

Although we have seen that the NHS was built on command and control that favoured transactional leadership there was a move over time towards a more transformational leadership approach with more clinical engagement and leadership at all levels (Budhoo and Spurgeon 2012). The leadership approach to management in the NHS of today is more humanistic and emotional and can even be a spiritual way of thinking according to Nicholson et al (2011) where, as stated previously, leaders and followers have an important role to play.

The NHS Outcomes Framework (2022) promotes a framework for all staff where they can build on best practice resulting in the reflective leader we will describe later in the book.

Table 1.1 is a summary of the effects of reports and reviews that have affected the changing approaches to healthcare leadership in the NHS.

Priorities for reform

Although we have seen these changes that have been made in the NHS we have also seen some reports of failures along the way that have affected leadership.

These include the:

- Allit Inquiry (Clothier et al 1994)
- Shipman (DoH 2004)
- Alder Hays Organs 1988–1995 (DoH 2001)
- Bristol Royal Infirmary children's Deaths in surgery (Bristol Royal Infirmary Inquiry 2001)
- Staffordshire Hospitals (Francis Report 2013).
- Morcambe Bay Hospitals (Kirkham Report 2015)
- Shrewsbury and Telford Hospitals (Ockenden Review 2022)

With leadership being intrinsically linked with patient care (Nicholson et al 2011) we need to continually strive to provide safe and effective care for all. This will mean using the appropriate approach at the appropriate time.

Table 1.1 Timeline of reports and reforms that have affected leadership and leaders within the NHS

Year	Main report/reform	Leadership style/changes
1948	Beven	Autocratic – 'great-man trait'
1962	Porritt Report	Situational – Single area board with doctor representation
1966	British medical Association Committee of inquiry into NHS	Situational – Representation of professions with doctor as chief officer
1967	Cogwheel report and Kings Fund/Institute of Hospital Administrators Joint Working Part	Distributed/situational approach – clear chain of command introduction of general managers
1972	Grey Book	Distributed – multidisciplinary approach
1973	NHS Reorganisation Act	Consensus – Devolution to smaller units- creation of regional and area health authorities.
1979 and 1980	Royal Commission and Health Service Act	Opposed to consensus – created district health authorities and smaller units
1983	Griffiths Report	Introduction of general managers
1989 and 1990	Working for Patients and NHS and Community Care Act	Creation of internal market and GPs purchasers of services.
1993 and 1995	Managing the new NHS and Health Authorities Act	Transformational – Regional health authorities abolished and creation of 8 regional offices.

Year	Policy/Document	Description
1999	Health Act	Transformational – Introduction of National Institute for Clinical Excellence and established Commission for Health Improvement. Removed GP fundholding
2000	NHS Plan	Competence – Performance targets
2004	NHS Leadership Qualities Framework	Built on medical competence framework
2008	Darzi report (NHS Next Stage Review)	Situational leadership – Greater emphasis on clinical leadership
2009	Inspiring Leaders: Leadership for Quality	Nurture potential talent
2010	Health and Social Care Bill; Liberating the NHS	Shifting accountability introducing national commissioning boards and local GP consortia. Regulated market and foundation status for trusts. Introduction of mutual and social enterprises.
2010	NHS Institute for Innovation and Improvement and Academy of Medical Royal Colleges: Clinical Leadership Competency Framework (CLCF)	All practising clinicians have a responsibility to strive to play a part in the leadership process and to encourage the leadership capacity of colleagues. The model in the CLCF is designed around 'delivering the service' and has five domains: 1 Demonstrating personal qualities 2 Working with others 3 Managing services 4 Improving services 5 Setting direction
2011	Kings Fund	Clear national focus of leadership shift towards autonomy, responsibility and accountability

(Continued)

Table 1.1 (Continued)

Year	Main report/reform	Leadership style/changes
2013	Berwick Report	'Board to bedside' to see care through patient's perspectives.
2013	Keogh review	Leadership at every level.
2013a	NHS Leadership Academy: Towards a new model of leadership:	includes technical competence, professional skills, managerial excellence, but care, compassion and genuine investment in staff is the key.
2013b	Leadership Academy- Healthcare model: the nine dimensions of leadership behaviour	More reflective – greater self-awareness, evaluating and sharing
2013	Francis Report	Safety at heart and central theme of leadership
2014	Duty of Candour	More bottom-up approach.
2016	NHS Leadership Framework	Building on best practice and all staff involved. Utilising different approaches to leadership
2018	Kings Fund and NHS Providers	Leadership in today's NHS, delivering the impossible
2022	The Health Foundation	Strengthening NHS management and leadership
2022	The Messenger Report	Leadership for a collaborative and inclusive future

References

Bamford-Wade, A, Moss, C (2010). Transformational leadership and shared governance: An action study. *Journal of Nursing Management*, 18, 815–821. 10.1111/j.1365-2834.2010.01134.x.

Barr, J, Dowding, L (2012). *Leadership in Health Care* (2nd ed.). London. Sage publishers.

Bass, BM (1981). *Stogdill's Handbook of Leadership* (2nd ed.). New York: Free Press.

Bass, BM (1985). *Leadership and Performance Beyond Expectations*. New York: Free Press.

Bennett, N, Wise, C, Woods, P, et al (2003) *Review of Distributed Leadership*. Nottingham. National College for School Leadership.

Blanken, R (2019). *8 common leadership styles*. The Centre for Association Leadership. Available at https://www.asaecenter.org/resources/articles/an_plus/2019/december/eight-leadership-styles-and-when-to-use-them (accessed on the 27/10/22).

Budhoo, M, Spurgeon, P (2012). Views and understanding of clinicians on the leadership role and attitude to coaching as a development tool for clinical leadership. *The International Journal of Clinical Leadership*, 17, 123–129.

Burns, JM (1978). *Leadership.* New York; London: Harper and Row.

Care Quality Commission (2015). *Regulation 20: Duty of Candour*. London: Care Quality Commission. https://www.cqc.org.uk/guidance-providers/all-services/regulation-20-duty-candour (Accessed 24/01/23).

Cardoso, MLAP, Ramos, LH, D'Innocenzo, M (2013). Coaching leadership: Leaders and followers' perceptions assessment questionnaires in nursing. *Einstein*, 12(1), 66–74.

Carroll, B, Levy, L, Richmond, D (2008). Leadership as practice: Challenging the competency paradigm. *Leadership*, 4, 363–379. 10.1177/1742715008095186.

Caulkins, DD (2008). Re-theorizing Jim Collins's culture of discipline in good to be great innovation. *The European Journal of Social Science Research*, 21(3), 217–232.

Chen, Cy, Chen, CHV, Li, CI (2013). The influence of leader's spiritual values of servant leadership of employee motivational autonomy and eudemonic well-being. *Journal of Religious Health*, 52(4), 418–438.

Clothier, C, MacDonald, C, Shaw, D (1994). Independent inquiry into deaths and injuries on the children's ward at Grantham and Kesteven General Hospital during the period February to April 1991 (Allitt Inquiry). London: Department of Health HMSO.

Cohen, WA (1990). *The Art of a Leader*. Englewood Cliffs, New Jersey: Jossey-Bass.

Collins, J (2001). *Good to be Great*. London: Random House Business.

Currie, G, Lockett, A, Suhomlinova, O (2009). The institutionalization of distributed leadership: A 'Catch-22' in English public services. *Human Relations*, 62(11), 1735–1761.

Davies, N (2013). Visible leadership: going back to the front line. *Nursing Management*, 20(40), 22–26. 10.7748/nm2013.07.20.4.22.e1086.

Downtown, JV (1973). *Rebel Leadership*. New York: Free Press.

de Zulueta, PC (2016). Developing compassionate leadership in health care: An integrative review. *Journal of Healthcare Leadership*, 8, 1–10.

Department of Health and Social Security (1972). *Management Arrangements for the Re-organised Health Service: The Grey Book*. London: HMSO. https://navigator.health.org.uk/theme/grey-book (Accessed 24/01/23).

Department of Health (1973). *NHS Reorganisation Act of 1973*. London: HMSO. http://www.legislation.gov.uk/ukpga/1973/32/pdfs/ukpga_19730032_en.pdf (Accessed 24/01/23).

Department of Health (1980). *Heath Services Act 1980*. London: HMSO. http://www.legislation.gov.uk/ukpga/1980/53/pdfs/ukpga_19800053_en.pdf (Accessed 24/01/23).

Department of Health (1989). *Working for Patients*. Cm 555. London: HMSO. https://navigator.health.org.uk/content/working-patients-1989 (Accessed 24/01/23).

Department of Health (1990). *NHS and Community Care Act*. London: HMSO. Available at http://www.legislation.gov.uk/ukpga/1990/19/contents/enacted (Accessed 24/01/23).

Department of Health (1993). *Managing the New NHS*. London: The Stationary Office.

Department of Health (1995). *Health Authority Act 1995*. London: HMSO. http://www.legislation.gov.uk/ukpga/1995/17/pdfs/ukpga_19950017_en.pdf (Accessed 24/01/23).

Department of Health (1999). *Health Act 1999*. London: HMSO. http://www.legislation.gov.uk/ukpga/1999/8/pdfs/ukpga_19990008_en.pdf (Accessed 24/01/23).

Department of Health (2000). *The NHS Plan. A Plan for Investment. A Plan for Reform*. London: DoH. http://webarchive.nationalarchives.gov.uk/20130124064356/http://www.dh.gov.uk/prod_consum_dh/groups/dh_digitalassets/@dh/@en/@ps/documents/digitalasset/dh_118522.pdf (Accessed 24/01/23).

Department of Health (2001). *The Royal Liverpool Children's Inquiry*. London: DoH. https://assets.publishing.service.gov.uk/government/uploads/system/uploads/attachment_data/file/250934/0012_ii.pdf (Accessed 23/01/23).

Department of Health (2004). *Shipman Inquiry Safeguarding Patients: Lessons from the Past – Proposals for the Future*. London. HMSO. http://webarchive.nationalarchives.gov.uk/20090808163837/http://www.the-shipman-inquiry.org.uk/5r_page.asp (Accessed 24/01/23).

Department of Health (2008). *High Quality Care for All: NHS 'Next Stage' Review Final Report*. London: The Stationery Office. Available at: http://webarchive.nationalarchives.gov.uk/20130107105354/http://www.dh.gov.uk/en/Publicationsandstatistics/Publications/PublicationsPolicyAndGuidance/DH_085825 (Accessed 24/01/23).

Department of Health (2009). *Inspiring Leaders: Leadership for Quality*. London: HMSO. http://webarchive.nationalarchives.gov.uk/20130124045141/http://www.dh.gov.uk/prod_consum_dh/groups/dh_digitalassets/documents/digitalasset/dh_093407.pdf (Accessed 24/01/23).

Department of Health (2010). *Equity and Excellence: Liberating the NHS*. London: The Stationery Office. https://assets.publishing.service.gov.uk/government/uploads/system/uploads/attachment_data/file/213823/dh_117794.pdf (Accessed 24/01/23).

Department of Health (2013). *Patients First and Foremost – The Initial Government Response to the Report of the Mid Staffordshire NHS Foundation Trust Public Inquiry*. London: The Stationery Office. https://assets.publishing.service.gov.uk/government/uploads/system/uploads/attachment_data/file/170701/Patients_First_and_Foremost.pdf (Accessed 24/01/23).

Department of Health and National Skills Academy for Social Care (2004). *Leadership Qualities Framework*. London: Department of Health and National Skills Academy for Social Care. https://www.skillsforcare.org.uk/Documents/Leadership-and-management/Leadership-Qualities-Framework/Leadership-Qualities-Framework.pdf (Accessed 24/01/23).

Department of Health and Social Care (2022). *Final Report of the Ockenden Review, GOV.UK*. GOV.UK. Available at: https://www.gov.uk/government/publications/final-report-of-the-ockenden-review (Accessed 24/01/23).

Department of Health and Social Security (1983). *NHS Management Inquiry. Griffiths Report on the NHS*. London: HMSO. https://www.sochealth.co.uk/national-health-service/griffiths-report-october-1983/ (Accessed 24/01/23).

Edmonstone, J (2013). What is wrong with the NHs Leadership development. *British Journal of Healthcare Management*, 19(110), 531–538.

Ellis, P, Abbot, J (2013). Leadership and management skills in health care. *British Journal of Cardiac Nursing*, 8(2), 96–99.

Elmore, RF (2004). *School Reform from the Inside Out: Policy, Practice, and Performance*. Cambridge, MA: Harvard Education Press.

Francis, R (2013). *Report of the Mid Staffordshire NHS foundation trust*. London: Public Inquiry. The Stationary Office.

Gill, R (2011). *Theory and Practice of Leadership* (2nd ed). London: Sage.

Goleman, D, Boyatzis, R, McKee, A (2002). *The New Leaders; Transforming the Art of Leadership into the Science of Results*. London: Sphere.

Greenleaf, RK (1970). *The Servant as Leader* cited by The Greenleaf Centre for servant leadership. Available at https://greenleaf.org/what-is-servant-leadership/ (accessed 27/10/22).

Greenleaf, RK (1991). *The Servant as Leader*. Indiana: The Robert K Greenleaf Centre for Servant Leadership.

Greenstein, J (2012). Level 5 leadership. *ACA News*, 24–25.

Gresh, MR (2006). Servant leadership a philosophical foundation for professionalism in physical therapy. *Journal of Physical Therapy Education*, 20(2), 12–16.

Grint, K (2005). Problems, problems, problems: The social construction of 'leadership'. *Human Relations*, 58(11), 1467–1494.

Hemphill, JK, Coons, AE (1957). Development of the leader behaviour description questionnaire. In Stodgill, RM, Coons, AE (Eds.) *Leader Behaviour: Its Description and Measurement*. Columbus, Ohio: Bureau of Business Research, Ohio State University, 6–38.

Hersey, P, Blanchard, K (1988). *Management of Organizational Behavior*. New Jersey, Englewood Cliffs: Prentice Hall.

Hollander, EP (1978). *Leadership Dynamics: A Practical Guide to Effective Relationships*. New York: Free Press.

Howard, G (1967). *The Shape of Hospital Management in 1980: The report of a Joint Working Party set up by the King's Fund and the Institute of Hospital Administrators*. London: King Edward's Hospital Fund for London and the Institute of Hospital Administrators.

Johnson, CE (2012). Meeting the Ethical Challenges of Leadership Casting Light or Shadow (4th ed). London: Sage.

Jones, L (2008). Leadership in the new NHS. *Nursing Management*, 15(16), 32–35.

Jones, L, Bennett, CL (2012). *Leadership in Health and Social Care, An Introduction for Emerging Leaders*. Banbury: Lantern Publishing Ltd.

Kotter, JP (2012). *Leading Change (with new preface)*. Boston: Harvard Business Review Press.

Kings Fund (2011). *The future of leadership and management in the NHS. No more heroes*. London: Kings Fund. https://www.kingsfund.org.uk/sites/default/files/future-of-leadership-and-management-nhs-may-2011-kingsfund.pdf (accessed 27/10/22).

Kings Fund (2-18) Leadership in today's NHS. Delivering the impossible. Available at: https://www.kingsfund.org.uk/sites/default/files/2018-07/Leadership_in_todays_NHS.pdf (accessed 29/10/22).

Kouzes, JM, Posner, BZ (1995). *The Leadership Challenge*. San Francisco: Jossey-Bass.

Leech, D (2012). Is a fresh prescription required for NHS leadership? *British Journal of Healthcare Management*, 18(11), 583.

Leigh, JA, Wild, J, Hynes, C et al (2014). Transforming community services through the use of a multidimensional model of clinical leadership. *Journal of Clinical Nursing*, 24, 749–760.

Lintern, S (2013). Hunt's US fast-track management scheme will cost £10 million. HSJ 26 September.

Mahon, K (2011). In praise of servant leadership horizontal service to others. *Canadian Association of Critical Care Nurses*, 22(4), 5–6.

McCombe, J (2013). Is current NHS leadership sufficient or deficient? *British Journal of Healthcare Management*, 19(7), 342–347.

McKimm, J, McLean, M (2020). Rethinking health professions' education leadership: Developing 'eco-ethical' leaders for a more sustainable world and future. *Medical Teacher*, 42(8), 855–860.

Michie, S, West, MA (2004). Managing people and performance: An evidence based framework applied to health service organizations. *International Journal of Management Reviews*, 5-6, 91–111. 10.1111/j.1460-8545.2004.00098.x.

Ministry of Health (1967). *First Report of the Joint Working Party on the Organisation of Medical Work in Hospitals (The Cogwheel Report)*. London: HMSO.

Ministry of Health and the Scottish Home and Health Department: *"medical manpower"* (1966) Wellcome collection. Available at: https://wellcomecollection.org/works/n8jjeqxa (Accessed: January 29, 2023).

Moll, S, Ahmed-Little, Y, Brown, B et al (2011). Emerging clinical leadership development in the NHS. *British Journal of Healthcare Management*, 17(10), 481–485.

Muls, A, Dougherty, L, Doyle, N et al (2015). Influencing organisational culture: A leadership challenge. *British Journal of Nursing*, 24(12), 633–638. 10.12968/bjon.2015.24.12.633.

NHS Digital (2022). NHS outcomes framework, NHS. Available at: https://digital.nhs.uk/data-and-information/publications/statistical/nhs-outcomes-framework/march-2022 (Accessed 24/01/23).

NHS England (2016). *Leading Change, Adding Value*. https://www.england.nhs.uk/wp-content/uploads/2016/05/nursing-framework.pdf (Accessed 24/01/23).

NHS England (2023). Our shared ambition for compassionate, inclusive leadership. https://www.england.nhs.uk/ourwork/part-rel/nqb/our-shared-ambition-for-compassionate-inclusive-leadership/ (Accessed 06/01/23).

NHS Improvements (2016). *Implementing the Forward View: Supporting Providers to Deliver*. https://assets.publishing.service.gov.uk/government/uploads/system/uploads/attachment_data/file/499663/Provider_roadmap_11feb.pdf (Accessed 24/01/23).

NHS Institute for Innovation and Improvement (2004). *NHS Leadership Qualities Framework: A Good Practice Guide*. Coventry: University of Warwick.

NHS Institute for Innovation and Improvement and Academy of Medical Royal Colleges (2010). Clinical Leadership Competency Framework (CLCF). https://www.leadershipacademy.nhs.uk/wp-content/uploads/2012/11/NHSLeadership-Leadership-Framework-Clinical-Leadership-Competency-Framework-CLCF.pdf (Accessed 24/01/23).

NHS Leadership Academy (2013a). Towards a new model of leadership. https://www.leadershipacademy.nhs.uk/wp-content/uploads/2013/05/ Towards-a-New-Model-of-Leadership-2013.pdf (Accessed 24/01/23).

NHS Leadership Academy (2013b). Healthcare leadership model: The nine dimensions of leadership. https://www.leadershipacademy.nhs.uk/ resources/healthcare-leadership-model/nine-leadership-dimensions/ (Accessed 24/01/23).

Nicholson, P, Rowland, E, Lokman, P et al (2011). *Leadership A Better Patient Care: Managing NHS*. London: HMSO.

Northouse, PG (2012). *Leadership: Theory and Practice* (5th ed). London: Sage.

Northouse, PG (2014). *Introduction to Leadership Concepts and Practice* (3rd ed). London: Sage.

Patel, VW, Warren, O, Humphris, P (2010). What does leadership in surgery entail? *ANZ Journal of Surgery*, 80, 876–883.

Porritt, A (1962). Report of the Medical Services Review Committee. *British Medical Journal*, 2, 1178–1186.

Porter-O'Grady, T, Malloch, K (2016). *The Leadership of Nursing Practice: Changing the Landscape of Health Care*. Cambridge, MA: Jones and Bartlett Learning.

Rauch, CF, Behling, O (1984). Functionalism: Basis for an alternate approach to the study of leadership. In Hunt, JG, Hosking, DM, Schriesheim, CA, Stewart, R (Eds.) *Leaders and Managers: International Perspectives on Managerial Behavior and Leadership*. New York: Pergamon Press, 45–62.

Schilling, J (2009). From ineffectiveness to destruction: A qualitative study on the meaning of negative leadership. *Leadership*, 5(1), 102–128.

Sherring, S (2012). Nursing leadership within the NHS: An evolutionary perspective. *British Journal of Nursing*, 21(8), 491–494.

Sofarelli, D, Brown, D (1998). The need of nursing leadership in uncertain times. *Journal of Nursing Management*, 6, 201–207.

Southworth, G (1998). *Leading Improving Primary Schools: The Work of Head Teachers and Deputy Head Teachers*. London: Falmer Press.

Stelter, R, Law, H (2010). Coaching narrative collaborative practice. *International Coaching Psychology Review*, 5(2), 152–164.

Stagecoach Group (2012). *South West Trains Managers Get Back to the Floor in Support of National Customer Service Week*. http://www.stagecoach. com/media/news-releases/2012/2012-10-05.aspx (Accessed 24/01/23).

Stogdill, RM (1950). Leadership, membership and organization. *Psychological Bulletin*, 47, 1–14.

Storey, J, Holti, R (2013). *Towards a New Model of Leadership in the NHS*. Available at https://www.leadershipacademy.nhs.uk/wp-content/uploads/ 2013/05/Towards-a-New-Model-of-Leadership-2013.pdf (Accessed on 27/10/22).

Thomas, H (2005). Clinical leadership: An oxymoron? *Clinician in Management*, 13, 111–114.

Thornton, P (2013). *Four Types of Leaders*. Available at http://www.trainingmag.com/four-types-leaders (Accessed on 27/10/22).

Waller, DJ, Smith, SR, Warnock, JT (1989). Situational theory of leadership. *American Journal of Health System Pharmacology*, 1(46), 2335–2341.

Warwick, P, Swaffield, S (2006). Articulating and connecting frameworks of reflective practice and leadership perspectives from 'fast track' trainee teachers. *Reflective Practice: International and Multidisciplinary Perspectives*, 7(2), 247–263.

Wasylyshyn, KM, Shorey, HS, Chaffin, JS (2012). Patterns of leadership behaviour: Implications for successful executive coaching outcomes. *The Coaching Psychologist*, 8(2), 74–85.

Waterman, H (2011). Principles of 'servant leadership' and how they can enhance practice. *Nursing Management*, 17(9), 24–26.

Watson, J et al. (2018). Quantum caring leadership: Integrating quantum leadership with caring science. *Nursing Science Quarterly*, 31(3), 253–258.

Yliruka, L, Karvinen-Niikoski, S (2013). How can we enhance the productivity in social work? Dynamically reflective structures, dialogue leadership and development of transformative expertise. *Journal of Social Work Practice*, 27(2), 191–206.

Chapter 2

What makes an excellent leader?

There is no one definition of a leader that fits all situations (Kings Fund 2011). If we look at the lists offered previously then it would seem that adopting a style and developing the characteristics is all it takes to be a good leader. However, if we are to measure a good leader by the quantitative output of productivity, or as Warwick and Swaffield (2006) point out what they do rather than the actions taken and the outcomes, then maybe that is as far as we need to go. However, this does not take into consideration the complex nature of healthcare today, the relationships and connections we have with our colleagues, the culture we help create around us, how we enable others to grow and how to help others to develop professionally. Therefore, rather than looking only at productivity, we need to take a more phenomenological, rather than just quantitative, approach to leadership beginning with self-awareness and reflection (Horton-Deutsch 2013). This, according to Stelter and Law (2010), is not something definite and final but is constructed in the present moment of experiencing and it changes from one situation to another. This in turn can result in a leader who thinks strategically with an integration of cognitive and emotional mental processing, through humanitarian collaboration and evolutionary processes and which embraces all those involved in the organisation (Looman 2003). This is from the employer and employee to those who access any of the services.

Bolden and Gosling (2006) also found that excellent leaders valued learning on the job and information from others whilst they constantly seek ways to improve practice.

Other arguments as to what makes an excellent leader have been in the nature-nurture debate. However, many writers believe that

DOI: 10.4324/9781003324560-2

there is no such thing as a born leader but that these skills and attributes are acquired early on in our lives. They suggest that through our early childhood and into adulthood it is our education, employment and life experiences that shape us as leaders and followers (Blanken 2019). However, as Jones and Bennett (2012) point out, some traits can be confused with being born a leader as when we review the list they may imply that some of those are traits that we are born with. Nonetheless, as they also point out, many of us are born with different traits that can also have an impact on our leadership approach and as Warwick and Swaffield (2006) agree, personal qualities do matter and can strongly influence actions and outcomes but are not the only factors in being a good leader. Recently there has also been a move to leader development rather than leadership development, as putting leadership into people has become less popular (Edmonstone 2013).

In this post 'heroic' period of leadership, leaders also need to understand that excellent leaders cannot be understood in the absence of their followers (Grint and Holt 2011). Leadership then should be centred on the vision and inspiration they impart on the people that they are working with to create a move towards the achievement of a common goal (Jones and Bennett 2012). The leader also needs to create a climate in which the individual acts to improve services and care within the NHS (Kings Fund 2011) whilst at the same time motivating others to fulfil that vision. This will include being inclusive, reflective and learning in real time (Quinn 2004), using emotional and social intelligence whereby the leader works more reflexively (Nicholson et al 2011). Therefore, the excellent leader must be mindful of their own practice and learn from it, whilst at the same time, being mindful of their followers and the organisation's needs and goals. Some of these aspects are discussed further within this part of the book as we review what makes an appreciative, ethical, positive and resonant leader.

Leadership that makes a difference

If our aim is to be a good leader and, at the same time, to create a supportive and developmental environment for those we work with, we need to increase our self-awareness. We need to identify with those traits, characteristics and styles and take responsibility for our impact on those we work with and start to think in different ways. As Louis R Mobley, the director of IBM's executive school in the 1950–1960s, stated *'leadership lives in how we think, not what we think'*. This *'radical revolution in consciousness'* that he spoke about is still relevant for today's leaders (cited in Blanken 2019). Therefore, this lends itself to a more critical appreciation of, and alternative approaches to, leadership for those working within healthcare. With the constant challenges, changes and complex nature of the healthcare service of the twenty-first century, the leader needs to adopt new approaches as well as be able to adapt their approach to leadership depending on the situation in which they find themselves. For example, on a busy surgical ward, on theatre day, the leader needs to be decisive and be able to bring a calming approach to the ward and staff working in it as opposed to the outpatient department where staff may become bored with routine and therefore this area requires a more dynamic creative leader to motivate and inspire the staff in their work.

Another aspect of leadership that makes a difference is the leader who looks below the surface. French and Bells (1990) developed their iceberg model of organisational culture where the tip, that is where the behaviour is demonstrated, is often the only area that causes a reaction. However, as Brown (2006) notes, it is what is happening below the waterline where we find the real dimensions of organisational life and it is this section of the iceberg that shapes what we see. These structures and behaviours can help us identify the mind-sets and see how people think. Brown (2006) also suggests that by reviewing this lower level the leader can influence the change of the mind-sets that affects everything above it.

Additionally, Knowles et al (2022) refer to the value of considering your purpose from a three-point aspect: social good, competence and culture in order to fine tune a clarity of purpose.

The appreciative leader

As part of the modern NHS and healthcare services the new paradigm of leadership calls for the leader to be a more appreciative leader.

This appreciative approach to leadership, according to Whitney and Trosten-Bloom (2011), requires a paradigm shift from the traditional, habitual and individualistic control and command practices towards a more positive style that involves socially generative principles, strategies and practices of appreciative leadership. Their definition of the appreciative leader is *'The relational capacity to mobilize creative potential and turn it into positive power – to set in motion positive ripples of confidence, energy, enthusiasm, and performance – to make a positive difference in the world.'* (Whitney and Trosten-Bloom 2011, p. 42). It is about the art of doing, according to Saiduddin et al (2009), who go on to suggest that this is about developing your own leadership style from the inside out which embraces the core appreciative inquiry principles.

Whitney and Trosten-Bloom (2011) also offer us five strategies for being an appreciative leader. These include:

- The wisdom of inquiry – asking positive powerful questions.
- The art of illumination – getting the best out of people.
- The genius of inclusion – by engaging with others to co create the future.
- The courage of inspiration – awaking our creative spirit.
- The path of integrity – making choices that are for the good of the whole.

The value of this approach to leadership also relies on our personal values including how we see ourselves as leaders, according to Schiller and Worthing (2011), and in doing that being able to gain a deeper appreciation of the people we work with and see where they are coming from (Whitney and Trosten-Bloom 2011). The language we use is also important and engaging in conversation with others is pivotal for this approach (Davy and Weiss 2011; Saiduddin et al 2009) as well as reflecting and building in moments of reflection (de Jong 2011), having a positive attitude (Lewis and Moore 2011; Schiller and Worthing 2011) being inclusive and celebrating practice (Lewis and Moore 2011), building on strengths rather than illuminating problems (Saiduddin et al 2009) and making things happen and creating energy (Schiller and Worthing 2011).

Ethical leader

Leaders can have an unusual degree of power and often they do not know they are making choices, or how to reflect on the process of making decisions, according to Johnson (2012). However, the ethical leader is aware of these and bases their leadership style on moral and ethical imperatives (Rucinski and Bauch 2006). They are concerned with perseverance, public spiritedness, integrity, truthfulness, fidelity, benevolence and humility (Rucinski and Bauch 2006). When we talk about ethical leaders, Rosenberg (2010) noted that we cannot disassociate it from reflective practice and happiness as they are all interrelated. However, as Johnson (2012) notes, there is also a darker and more negative dimension to leadership that can be destructive. Therefore Johnson (2012) suggests that leaders need to take into consideration the ethical burdens such as power, privilege, information, consistency, loyalty and responsibility. Through the handling of these, he suggests, we can do harm as well as good, therefore the ethical leader needs to be involved in new roles of engagement that include reflective thinking, ethical and moral behaviour with a commitment to social justice (Rucinski and Bauch 2006) in order to do good rather than harm. Warwick and Swaffield (2006) noted that moral purposes must have active concerns for the aims and consequences in relation to making a positive difference to those in the workplace as well as to society as a whole. Northouse (2012) then suggests that an ethical leader is one that is grounded in the concept of duty and personal responsibility. These leaders include the values of the workforce, organisation and community in which they work. He went onto suggest that there are two domains of ethical leadership theory, these include the conduct and character of the leader and secondly the actions and consequences of those actions. Ethical leadership, he suggests, is about who the person is as an individual. These virtues and morals of being an ethical leader are not innate but can be learnt according to Rucinski and Bauch (2006). The ethical leader is grounded in their own values and should have confidence in their self-knowledge with an ability to grow and change (Northouse 2012). Recent research has indicated that in times of crisis, an ethical leader is likely to speak out against wrong doing or inequity (Musbahi et al 2022).

Starratt (1991) also included three themes when referring to the conduct of an ethical leader which are critique, justice and caring. Shapiro and Stefkovich (2003) agree and produced four similar themes of; ethics of justice, critique, care and profession. Whilst Rucinski and Bauch (2006) summarised that this approach should involve a move away from the bureaucratic systems and control and that there should be a focus on empowerment and participatory decision making within the team.

However, in healthcare, there is a legal and political framework that defines our work and, as Wright (2009) points out, this must be reflected in the moral purposes and relationship between policy and practice which can, in turn, lead to significant dilemmas for the ethical leader.

This ethical leadership approach is therefore very much based on the relationship and participatory approach promoted by the authors of this book.

Positive leader

The positive leader, according to Tombaugh (2005), demonstrates traits such as optimism, self-confidence, compassion, emotional intelligence, loyalty and trustworthiness. These leaders, they go on to suggest, promote a strengths-based organisation that is based on possibilities where they maintain a committed and motivated workforce that is open to learning and growth rather than the traditional problem-solving/deficit-based approach. It is the relationship with their staff that, according to Stichler (2009), is one of the greatest factors in developing a positive and healthy work environment. This involves a caring leader that is authentic and who is aware of how they think and behave, as well as how they are perceived by others (Uusaiutti 2013). They also have a long-term vision that is embedded in creating meaningful work with a positive outlook (Kaipa and Kriger 2010) and can be clearly articulated so that it influences others to follow (Stichler 2009).

Resonant leader

In a time of change, budget cuts and endless reorganisations, the leader needs to show empathy and be attuned to people's feelings, being able to move them in a positive emotional direction (Goleman et al 2002a). This can, according to Goleman et al (2002a), be developed through the resonant leader, a sub-category of transformational leader, who in times of stress is able to listen to the workers, provide empathy whilst being supportive and building a positive work climate and increase the emotional health of the workforce. Goleman et al (2002a) also state that being a resonant leader incorporates self-assessment with the ability to accurately perceive one's own performance. This approach is embedded and relies on a degree of emotional intelligence (Goleman et al 2002a, 2002b; Lutzo 2005; Watson 2014). The characteristics of this leader include; the ability to maintain a productive relationship, ability to cultivate mindfulness, show compassion, instil hope whilst aligning skills and relationships with the goals of the team (Lutzo 2005; Watson 2014). They should be able to connect with others (Goleman et al 2002b) whilst being upbeat and having enthusiastic energy, being collaborative with emotional bonds where ideas are shared, learning occurs from each other, people's feelings are understood and they are cared for (Goleman et al 2002a). Being able to imagine a better and feasible future even in times of change is also a key skill (Lutzo 2005).

This approach to leadership involves building on the skills we already possess such as empathy whilst using a more strength based and positive approach to leadership as noted above.

Authentic leader

This approach was introduced to address the more turbulent workplace seen in recent years. Based in the positive school of psychology, the authentic leader central premise is through increased self-awareness, self-regulation and positive modelling as a leader (Avolio and Gardner 2005). The leader is honest with oneself, sincere with others and their leadership approach should reflect their own personal values (Avolio et al 2004; Leroy et al 2015). It is through this approach that they can influence their followers with a focus on wellbeing (Avolio and Gardner 2005). It is through the enacting of being true to self that the authentic leader is transparent and behaves in an ethical manner that provides an open sharing of information with others. However, critics of this approach note that the studies in relation to the authentic leader approach are too positive and that the fundamental theoretical approaches are flawed and require further serious scholarly enterprises and less ideological research (Alvesson and Einola 2019).

Conclusion

Leadership is affected by change and as a result of the changes new leadership approaches emerge. Having reviewed the different approaches styles and traits of a leader in the NHS over the decades since its inception we can start to see how the approaches have changed over time from the autocratic to the bureaucratic, transformational leader. However, the newer paradigms of leadership approach can help to develop a strengths-based, reflective leader that is able to adapt their leadership approach to the situation whilst supporting and developing others and valuing the role of the follower. This can in turn prevent some of the poorer outcomes of care seen in some of the reports and inquires noted within this chapter.

References

Alvesson, M, Einola, K (2019). Warning for excessive positivity: Authentic leadership and other traps in leadership studies. *The Leadership Quarterly*, 30(4), 383–395.

Avolio, BJ, Gardner, WL (2005). Authentic leadership development: Getting to the root of positive forms of leadership. *The Leadership Quarterly*, 16, 315–338.

Avolio, BJ, Gardner, WL et al (2004). Unlocking the mask: A look at the process by which authentic leaders impact follower attitudes and behaviours. *The Leadership Quarterly*, 15, 801–823.

Blanken, R (2019). *8 Common Leadership Styles*. The Centre for Association Leadership. Available at https://www.asaecenter.org/resources/articles/an_plus/2019/december/eight-leadership-styles-and-when-to-use-them (accessed on the 27/10/22).

Bolden, R, Gosling, J (2006). Leadership competencies: Time to change the tune? *Leadership*, 2(2), 147–163.

Brown, JS (2006). Reflective practices for transformational leaders. *Future Age*, 6–9. https://leadershipsaskatoon.com/resources/1314resources/

reflective%20practices%20for%20the%20transformational%20leader.pdf (Accessed 29/10/22).

Davy, JM, Weiss, LS (2011). Appreciative leadership in the face of tragedy. *AI Practitioner*, 13(1), 7–10.

De Jong, JC (2011). The daily disciplines and practices of an appreciative leader. *AI Practitioner*, 13(1), 22–23.

Edmonstone, J (2013). What is wrong with the NHs Leadership development. *British Journal of Healthcare Management*, 19(110), 531–538.

French, WL, Bells, CH (1990). *Organisation Development; Behavioural Science Interventions for Organisational Improvement* (4th ed). Harlow: Prentice Hall.

Goleman, D, Boyatzis, R, McKee, A (2002a). *The New Leaders; Transforming the Art of Leadership into the Science of Results*. London: Sphere.

Goleman, D, Boyatzis, R, McKee, A (2002b). *Primal Leadership*. Boston MA: Harvard Business School Press.

Grint, K, Holt, C (2011). *Followership in the NHS: A report for The King's Fund Commission on Leadership and Management in the NHS* [online]. Available at: https://www.kingsfund.org.uk/sites/default/files/followership-in-nhs-commississon-on-leadership-Management-keith-grint-claire-holt-kings-fund-may-2011.pdf (accessed 29/10/22).

Horton-Deutsch, S (2013). Thinking through the path to reflective leadership. *American Nurse Today*, 8(2).

Johnson, CE (2012). *Meeting the Ethical Challenges of Leadership Casting Light or Shadow* (4th ed). London: Sage.

Jones, L, Bennett, CL (2012). *Leadership in Health and Social Care, An Introduction for Emerging Leaders*. Banbury: Lantern Publishing Ltd.

Kaipa, P, Kriger, M (2010). Empowerment, vision and positive leadership. An interview with Alan Mulally former CEO Boeing commercial – current CEO Ford Motoring Company. *Journal of Management Inquiry*, 19(2), 110–115.

Kings Fund (2011). *The Future of Leadership and Management in the NHS. No More Heroes*. London: Kings Fund. https://www.kingsfund.org.uk/sites/default/files/future-of-leadership-and-management-nhs-may-2011-kings-fund.pdf (accessed 27/10/22).

Knowles, J, Hunsaker, BT, Grove, H, et al (2022 Mar/Apr). What is the purpose of your purpose? *Harvard Business Review*. Available at https://hbr.org/2022/03/what-is-the-purpose-of-your-purpose (Accessed it 10/04/23).

Leroy, H, et al (2015). Authentic leadership, authentic followership, basic need satisfaction and work role performance: A cross-level study. *Journal of Management*, 41(69), 1677–1697.

Lewis, S, Moore, L (2011). Positive and appreciative leadership. *AI Practitioner*, 13(1), 4–6.

Looman, MD (2003). Reflective leadership strategic planning from heart and soul. *Consulting Psychology Journal Practice and Research*, 5(4), 215–221.

Lutzo, E (2005). Resonant Leadership. *Weatherhead School of Management Alumni Association*, 2(11), 1.

Mobley, L cited in Blanken, R (2019). *8 Common Leadership Styles*. The Centre for Association Leadership. Available at https://www.asaecenter.org/resources/articles/an_plus/2019/december/eight-leadership-styles-and-when-to-use-them (Accessed on the 27/10/220).

Musbahi, A, McCulla, A, Ramsingh, J (2022). Pandemic priorities: the impact of the COVID 19 pandemic on ethical leadership in the healthcare profession. *Leadership in Health Services*, 35(4), 506–518. 10.1108/LHS-02-2022-0011.

Nicholson, P, Rowland, E, Lokman, P et al (2011). *Leadership A Better Patient Care: Managing NHS*. London; HMSO.

Northouse, PG (2012). *Leadership: Theory and Practice* (5th ed). London: Sage.

Quinn, RE (2004). *Building the Bridge as You Walk on It: A Guide for Leading Change*. San Francisco: Jossey-Bass.

Rosenberg, LR (2010). Transforming leadership: Reflective practice and the enhancement of happiness. *Reflective Practice*, 11(1), 9–18.

Rucinski, DA, Bauch, PA (2006). Reflective ethical and moral constructs in educational leadership preparation: Effects on graduates' practice. *Journal of Educational Administration*, 44(5), 487–508.

Saiduddin, MH, Larrson, S, Lundqvist, M (2009). Appreciative leadership. An insider's perspective on changing reality. *AI Practitioner*, 11(4), 4–8.

Schiller, MR, Worthing, L (2011). A decade of appreciative leadership thoughts and reflections. *AI Practitioner*, 13(1), 17–21.

Shapiro, JP, Stefkovich, JA (2003). *Ethical Leadership and Decision Making: Applying Theoretical Perspectives to Complex Dilemmas*. NJ: Lawrence Erlbaum Associates.

Starratt, RJ (1991). Building an ethical school: A theory for practice in educational leadership. *Educational Administration Quarterly*, 27(2), 185–202.

Stelter, R, Law, H (2010). Coaching narrative collaborative practice. *International Coaching Psychology Review*, 5(2), 152–164.

Stichler, JF (2009). Creating a healthy positive work environment. As leadership imperative. *Nursing for Women's Health*, 341–346.

Tombaugh, JR (2005). Positive leadership yields performance and profitability; effective organizations develop their strengths. *Development and Learning Organizations. An International Journal*, 19(3), 15–17.

Uusaiutti, S (2013). An action orientated perspective on caring leadership a qualitative study of higher education administrators positive leadership experiences. *International Journal of Leadership in Education Theory and Practice*, 16(4), 482–496.

Warwick, P, Swaffield, S (2006). Articulating and connecting frameworks of reflective practice and leadership perspectives from 'fast track' trainee teachers. *Reflective Practice: International and Multidisciplinary Perspectives*, 7(2), 247–263.

Watson, R (2014). Twenty-first century management: Resonant leadership and emotional intelligence. *ACA News*, 36.

Whitney, D, Trosten-Bloom, A (2011). Five strategies of Appreciative leadership. *AI Practitioners*, 13(1), 41–43.

Wright, LL (2009). Leadership in the swamp: Seeking the potentiality of school improvement through principle reflection. *Reflective Practice: International and Multidisciplinary Perspectives*, 10(2), 259–272.

Chapter 3

Linking leadership with reflection, reflexivity and action, putting our values into practice

Reflective leadership

With all the different approaches to leadership noted in the first part of this book, we may ask what has the reflective leader got to offer healthcare, the people that work in it and the organisation that the other approaches cannot offer? Although we have seen how leadership approaches have changed over the past decades in an attempt to meet the changing needs of the healthcare service we have not reached a situation where 'business as usual' is effective. The healthcare service continues to change and now at a faster pace than ever before. A new significant challenge that we are currently facing is that there is a need for a clear focus to balance cost whilst at the same time providing high-quality service improvements (Darzi 2008; DoH 2010; Francis 2013; Keogh 2013; NHS England 2016; NHS Improvement 2016), and this whilst moving through a prolonged time of austerity in funding, with an increased focus from regulators, politicians and the media (Kings Fund 2018). In the light of the impact of the COVID-19 pandemic on healthcare organisation and delivery, there is a further imperative to make savings (Anderson 2022). In order to meet these, we need leaders who can utilise the best of the leadership approaches noted earlier but also to develop a more collective and supportive approach to leadership that adapts to change and at the same time develops the leaders of the future. We therefore argue that the reflective leader can address these challenges in a changing environment noted whilst at the same time developing future leaders. These leaders can also help to improve the self-esteem,

DOI: 10.4324/9781003324560-3

confidence and standards of wellbeing of the people that they work with, help to identify meaningful solutions and decisions that are embedded in evidence-based practice with goal clarity and develop a collaborative team approach that assists the continual professional development and learning of all the participants.

We need to remind ourselves that leadership is a journey rather than a destination, a process rather than an event, continuous rather than episodic, unpredictable and is required to survive, as suggested by Schwahn and Spady (1998), it is not something that we learn and do and move on from and this therefore fits with the reflective leader approach.

This part of the book will help us understand the difference and similarities to other leadership styles noted in the first part of the book that can help the reflective leader to use the most appropriate approaches. It will review some of the terms used associated with levels and types of reflection and reflexivity for the leader and how we can use these in leadership roles whilst creating a reflective practice environment that meets the growing demands and challenges of the service. Finally, it will discuss ways that we can put our values in to practice as a reflective leader using our emotional intelligence, appreciative intelligence and narrative intelligence.

Reflection in leadership

This approach draws on many of the characteristics of the ethical, appreciative and positive leader noted previously but develops these further to meet the new and changing needs of the developing healthcare service. Using reflection is not unique to the reflective leader and is seen in other approaches including change management and transformational leadership theories. However, for the reflective leader there is a greater emphasis on reflection that requires thinking more critically and reflexively about ourselves, the team, all of our actions and the situations in which we find ourselves within the organisation in which we work (Cunliffe 2009). This is more than a self-reflection that we often use for our continuing professional development as required by our professional bodies. It involves including others in the team as we all search for compassionate consideration about any problems encountered (Göker and Bozkuş 2017), is rooted in evidence-based knowledge where theory and practice come together and includes a collective act of joint and careful thinking (Ekebergh 2001) and long-term planning and finding intuitive ways to solve problems (Castelli 2016).

Through this process we can increase the likelihood of product success by addressing the challenges of balancing some of the cost-, efficient service verses higher quality of care. We can do this through developing meaningful solutions and decisions that are embedded in evidence-based practice with goal clarity and increasing our under-standing of obstacles and how to address them with a forward action plan. Respecting each other including diverse cultures and customs and increasing personal and professional development and an interest in learning is also part of this role as a reflective leader. Lastly, being open and challenging our own and others beliefs and assumptions will help with team learning and new understanding where open conver-sations and dialogue are valued and team members are active in decision making. This is supported by many authors who have found that the values of a reflective approach to leadership: improves or-ganisational performance (Castelli 2016), helps with making decisions in ambiguous, unstable and unique situations (Rucinski and Bauch 2006), can affect other people's thinking (Jonasson et al 2017), de-velops future leaders (Castelli 2016), can provide significant oppor-tunities for learning and development (Matsuo 2016), avoids the knee-jerking/quick fix approach (Looman 2003) and produces a motivated workforce which renews interest and effort in work (Castelli 2016).

Defining reflection

Whilst reflection is a term that is widely used within healthcare, mainly in relation to continuing professional development or following adverse events, there are many definitions in the literature.

The definitions of reflection originate with the work of Dewey (1933) stating that it is an; *'active, persistent and careful consideration of any belief or supposed form of knowledge in the light of the grounds that support it and the further conclusion to which it tends'* and Schön (1983) *who states that it is 'questioning the assumptional structures of knowing-in-action' and thinking 'critically about that thinking that got us to fix this opportunity'*. *This has been followed by more* recent definitions such as Moon (1999, 2004) who stated it was a *'form of mental processing with a purpose and/or anticipated outcome that is applied to relatively complex or unstructured ideas for which there is not an obvious solution'*, and Kember (2000, 2008) who stated that *'reflection and critical reflection are viewed as two levels on a four-scale continuum of reflective thinking reflection'*, *'operates through a careful re-examination and evaluation of experience, beliefs and knowledge'* and *'leads to new perspectives'*; *critical reflection, the highest level of reflection, 'involving perspective transformation'* and *'necessitates a change to deep-seated, and often unconscious, beliefs and leads to new belief structures'*. Mann et al in 2009 stated that it is a *'purposeful critical analysis of knowledge and experience, in order to achieve deeper meaning and understanding'* and Sandars (2009) *'A metacognitive process that occurs before, during and after situations with the purpose of developing greater understanding of both the self and the situation so that future encounters with the situation are informed from previous encounters'*.

In 2014 after careful consideration of the previous definitions, Ngugen et al (2014, p. 1182) came up with their definition that *'reflection is the process of engaging the self in attentive, critical, exploratory and iterative interactions with one's thoughts and actions, and their underlying conceptual frame, with a view to changing them and with a view on the change itself'*.

Whilst the fundamental concept of reflection has not altered over the years with the definitions noted above, Kolb (1984) reminds us that reflection is a process and not an outcome and therefore as a reflective leader one of the main characteristics is that it is a continual activity. This is one the leader builds on to meet the challenges that are ahead as well as those we currently face.

Dixon et al (2016) also note the danger that we can become embroiled in Dewey (1933) and Schön (1983) original concepts of reflection and therefore we should not see reflection as a singular or uncontested term as this may limit our understanding and/or application of reflection to our practice, especially as reflective leaders. This is also noted in later definitions above; however, other authors argue that it should also not be restricted to ebbing a process of quiet self-fulfilment (Gray 2007) or as Matsuo (2016) notes, not just to refer to stepping back and pondering on the meaning of experiences to improve practice. This reflection, these authors argue, may restrict reflection to the past events and limit its use for the individual and reflective leader for present and future decision making. We need a wider approach to reflection that involves not just self but is also collaborative and includes reflection from practice, in practice and prior to practice.

Reflective approaches

As noted above, reflection is more than a personal action, it is a continual process (Kolb 1984) and is a conscious and intentional examination of our behaviour (Göker and Bozkuş 2017), and provides us with opportunities for us to re-evaluate what has been achieved in practice as well as identifying what improvements we could make incorporating a forward approach to practice and decision making (Göker and Bozkuş (2017). Therefore, there are different approaches to reflection, whilst we recognise the reflecting on past experiences and events, as often seen in the literature and described by Schön (1983, p. 87) as reflection-on-action. Schön (1983, p. 87) also referred to 'reflection-in-practice', the here and now and Van Manen (1995) talks about 'anticipatory' reflection or as Oeij et al (2017) called it 'ante-action-reflection' thinking and planning for practice before the event takes place.

Reflection-on-action is far more accepted within healthcare and tends to be where practitioners focus their actions/behaviours and involves thinking about past experiences and events that have already occurred. It is often required by professional bodies such as the Health and Care Professional Council and Nursing and Midwifery Council for practitioners to identify their continuing professional development and learning (Jonasson et al 2017). Therefore, this reflection is familiar within healthcare and whilst we recognise that there is a place for *'reflection on action'* as in Schön (1983, p. 87) and Dewey's (1933) work Göker and Bozkuş (2017) reminds us that these original authors for reflection both come from a problem-solving approach. This is reflected in many of the reflective models'that we often use such as Gibbs (1988), Johns (2004), Atkins and Murphy (1994), and others. The idea of 'fixing', as stated by Schön (1983), can lead us to mainly viewing reflection as coming from practice that has gone wrong, taking a negative orientation resulting in attempting to 'improve practice'.

The reflection-on-action in this situation is often a deliberate and cognitive process that is triggered by doubt, mental difficulty and hesitation where the problem activates reflection in order to find a solution to the current situation (Göker and Bozkuş 2017). This negative stance is further emphasised in the use of the term 'critical incident' as originally used by John Flannagan in 1954 and introduced into nursing by Benner in 1984 which Ghaye and Lillyman (2008) suggest in healthcare tends to conjure up thoughts of major and/or negative events. As Dixon et al (2016) point out, there is little suggestion that a positive event, where we seek to understand something in practice as the catalyst for reflection, is undertaken as much as negative events.

If we take this negative stance then, as Dixon et al (2016) noted, this can result in our reflection gravitating towards problems within the organisation or errors of individuals rather than a more positive approach to decision making and action planning. This can also result in the blame culture that can make leadership roles become less attractive to people within the organisation (Kings Fund 2018).

Whilst there is a place for reflection-on-action when practice does not go to plan there needs to be a balance with celebrating the positive aspects of practice to enhance future performance through reflection-on-action (Dixon et al 2016). Fredrickson (2003) and Fredrickson and Losada (2008) state that a 3:1 ratio of positive to negative thoughts is a good model for use. Using reflection on positive events and experiences several authors note how this positivity changes how our minds work and is related to positive engagement, reduced staff turnover, and enhanced productivity, performance and profitability (Dixon et al 2016; Isen and Labroo 2003; Fredrickson 2009) and that when people experience positive feelings, they are more flexible, creative, integrative, open to information and efficient in their thinking. Fredrickson (1998, 2001, 2004) reported in her broaden-and-build theory, that how we feel links us with what we can do, this she argues promotes positivity suggesting that when we feel positive then we are more receptive to new ideas, more adaptive and more adaptable and open minded. This approach also helps to build on the individual's personal resources and ability to build resistance which can be drawn on by the leader/managers within organisations and therefore an important tool for us as reflective leaders. Dixon et al (2016) also elaborate by stating that by drawing on skilled practice, using our positive experience, our knowledge and inquiry processes can increase our capability to intervene, interpret and act positively, gaining understanding of the root causes of success and to then be able to apply this to continue to develop our future performance.

Schön (1983, p. 87) in his work moved beyond thinking about past events to what he referred to as 'reflection-in-practice'. Here he suggests reflection can happen simultaneously with the event. This can be when we find ourselves in a situation when there is no time to step back and think about what we can do, or ahead of what might happen. This could be in a time-critical event or emergency situation. Whilst simultaneously acting we need to think about our actions, be aware of the situation we find ourselves in and use our experience and knowledge as best we can in that situation using mindfulness. Schon (1983) also notes that reflection-in-action can include on-the-spot reflective conversations which can help with the process of critically reviewing the situation, restructuring the process and even testing our initiative understanding of experiences phenomena during the event.

Anticipatory or ante-action-reflection as noted by Van Manen (1995) and Oeij et al (2017) is when we take time to reflect on potential situations and plan for these events before they happen. For example, our first day after qualifying in our professional role or taking on a new role we think long and hard before going to work, what might happen? We question to ourselves what will I do if this or that happens? How will I react to this or that? This reflection is taking place before the event has happened, our action plans are made in order for us to deal with the situation should it arise and these can play an important role as a reflective practitioner and leader, we cannot always wait for experiences or events but need time as well to prepare for events to occur where action plans are in place to deal with them as they arise.

For any form of reflection to occur, in, on or before, we must be engaged in a consistent practice of reflection (Castelli 2016). This involves a conscious awareness of our behaviours, situations and consequences with the ultimate aim of improving organisational performance and providing a quality service that is fit for practice (Castelli 2016).

Reflection therefore should become our work-based habit and part of our everyday process becoming a normal part of us and when working with colleagues and teams should become part of every member of the team's everyday work practice (Jonasson et al 2017).

Another approach that has been mentioned at times in this section is that of the team approach to reflection which originated with Tom Anderson et al (1987) in psychology. As reflective leaders, we need to create an environment where reflection needs to become a workplace habit that can, according to Ghaye (2011), over time develop into a reflective organisation. All personnel are dependent on each other for prompting care improvement within the organisation and therefore the reflective leader needs to develop this interpersonal mutual involvement (Jonasson et al 2014). This involves an act of joint reflection which Göker and Bozkuş (2017) and Jonasson et al (2014) all argue that professional competence that has often been unarticulated can become articulated and which, according to Stroebel et al (2005), leads to both a successful vision and learning for all concerned. Matsuo (2016) agrees that this team approach to reflection can provide significant opportunities for learning and development. In turn, this can develop a sense of togetherness, mutual respect and results in making it easier to set common goals that are congruent with professional values (Jonasson et al 2014). These include a supportive relationship (Castelli 2016; Herold et al 2008) where Looman (2003) highlights the importance of integrating human potential rather than splintering it. It is these good quality relationships and team approach to reflection that can result in good outcomes (Göker 2012). As a reflective leader, Göker (2012) goes on to suggest that creating this team approach requires self-reflection with a leadership that has an understanding about the organisational activities, shared purposes and goals.

Approaches to reflection, therefore, include before, after and during our practice and include both individual and team approaches. It is a continual process that needs to be facilitated in leaders and teams if we are to meet the changing needs and requirements of the healthcare service in which we work.

Levels of reflection

So, whilst as reflective leaders we can reflect on, in and/or before action we need to be aware of the different terms used to identify the type and levels of reflection noted within the literature. These include terms such as 'descriptive', 'critical', 'intense' and 'deep' reflection.

Descriptive reflection is usually the initial stage where we think about the event that has happened. It is often the start of many of the reflective models as discussed by Ghaye and Lillyman (2006). By putting the experience into words, or thoughts, at this stage it can be elevated and compared with previous experiences, leads onto further critical reflection (Jonasson et al 2017), often focuses on the immediate presenting details of a task or problem (Reynolds 1998) and is a conscious act of careful thinking (Ekebergh 2001). Whilst this level of reflection is important any reflection needs to be followed by action (Rucinskis and Bauch 2006). It is the act of reflection that makes possible the determination of an individual, team's and organisation's best course of action (Castelli 2016). However, the action then needs to be based on the research and evidence base that uses a wider perspective that then stimulates further reflection and development (Jonasson et al 2014). This leads us to the critical reflection seen below to take this process forward to become affective in practice.

'*Critical reflection*' (White et al 2006) or '*intensive reflection*' (Peltier et al 2005) are terms used and defined by Reynolds (1998) as the stage where there is an analysis of the power and control with an examination of the taken for granted within the task or problem situated. The terms critical, intensive and deep are often used interchangeably within the literature and models of reflection. It follows the descriptive reflection noted above and, as Reynolds (1998) argues, critical reflection is concerned with questioning assumptions, where it focuses on social rather than the individual and is concerned with emancipation. Gray (2007) goes on to suggest that critical reflection also raises questions that are moral as well as technical in nature and agrees that it must be a social act of collaborative empowerment.

Critical or deep reflection is a model of transformative learning where we alter our cognitive schema underlying our perspective on a specific subject (Mezirow 1991). Whilst Peltier et al (2005) suggested that *intensive reflection* is positively related to programme outcomes whereas habitual and understanding were negatively related to these outcomes.

It is through this critical/intensive or deep reflection, as a reflective leader, we are able to fill the gap between theory and practice by constructing our own theories of practice during, after and even before our action at the same time identifying and questioning any assumptions about practice (Sullivan and Weissner, 2010), learn from our previous events and experiences and identify why people reacted and/ or performed as they did in the given situations.

Through this level of reflection, we can also make informed decisions for future events moving informed practice forward. However, Gray (2007) notes that leaders do not necessarily automatically engage with critical reflectivity and therefore it is a skill that must be developed.

Whilst the authors above explain the difference between reflection and critical/intensive reflection other authors have broken the stages down further into different levels of reflection.

For example, Kember et al (2000) identified four levels of reflection:

- Habitual action
- Understanding
- Reflection
- Intensive reflection/critical

Whilst Goodman (1984 cited in Jasper 2003, p. 7) identified three levels of:

- descriptive
- connections of principles and
- practice through to a deeper level able to explore complex situations in depth by drawing on various theoretical, ethical, political, personal and professional perspectives

Rolfe et al (2001, pp. 34–36) also use three levels but identify these as a cyclical process of analysis that ranges from descriptive, theory building to an action-orientated stage. They also suggest that reflection can vary in depth at each stage. However with all these levels noted by the authors, the majority of models of reflection tend to start with description and build up to the deeper level suggesting that the last stage is where we have reached the critical/intensive level discussed earlier which in turn leads to learning and action planning.

Kemmis (1985) emphasised that although reflection is a mental process it should also be a social action. The social aspect is evident in some of the other authors noted above together with authors such as Reynolds (1999), Horton-Deutsch (2013) and Jonasson et al (2017) who all emphasise the collective team approach to reflection, as discussed earlier.

Göker and Bozkuş (2017) remind us reflection at any level is a vital and inherent component of the leader's everyday life affecting our choices, policies and decisions together with the emotions and politics related to them.

Reflexivity and the reflective leader

The terms reflection and reflexivity are often used interchangeably; however, the use and term of reflexivity dates back more than a century (Wendel et al 2018) and has been defined by many authors. Gray (2007) argues that reflexivity is very different from reflection which can be regarded as a modernist idea that searches for patterns, logic and order. In contrast, he quotes Cunliffe (2004) who states that reflexivity involves 'complexifying thinking or experiences by exploring contradictions, doubts, dilemmas and possibilities' (p. 505) and argues that it embraces subjective understanding or reality in order to think more critically about values and effect of one's actions on others.

In order to understand its concept, Goodman et al (1998, p. 273) provide us with a definition of reflexivity stating that it is a *'lived activity and reflection within one's community for the purpose of challenging assumptions and creating change toward the core public health values of democratic participation and equity'*. Whilst Rosenberg (1990, p. 3) stated that it is a process *'among human beings is rooted in the social process, particularly the process of taking the role of the other and of seeing the self from the other's perspective'*. Matsuo (2016) suggests that reflexivity is the extent to which an individual overtly reflects on his or her experience and, as suggested by Castelli (2016), is a conscious activity of purposeful reflection which is a process that requires critical thinking and problem-solving skills. Mezirow

(1991) sums it up and states that reflexivity ultimately leads to a change in behaviour and thus in outcomes.

All the authors noted the use of reflection as an active process which challenges assumptions and has a social context. Therefore, reflexivity requires reflection and by also being reflexive it can result in 'reflective practice' at an individual, team or organisational level. Cressey et al (2006) note that productive reflection conditions require collective rather than individual orientation. Carter and West (1998 cited in Dayan and Basarir 2008) also noted that the concept of reflexivity emerged as a key determinant of the performance of teams and that it is assumed to help teams know their actual workings and develop new understandings and methods that respond to emerging conditions and challenges.

Team reflexivity is also defined as 'the extent to which group members overtly reflect upon the group's objectives, strategies and processes, and adapt them to current and anticipated endogenous or environmental circumstances' (West 1996, p. 559 in Dayan and Basarir (2008). Team reflexivity naturally fits into disciplines aimed at individual problem-solving or self-improvement (Mezirow 1991), impacts on team performance (Dayan and Basarir 2008), facilitates team learning (Jonasson et al 2017; Boud et al 2006; Kolb 1984; Schon 1983; and West 1996) and the development of employees' creative problem-solving capacity (Carmeli et al 2013).

This team approach to reflexivity, whereby team reflexivity as argued by Dayan and Basarir (2008), can have an impact on team performance is contingent on environmental conditions. They suggest that when technology and markets are more predictable the team reflexivity on new produce success will be less but when technology and market are not predictable the impact of team reflexivity on new produce success will be higher. Therefore, this is appropriate to the ever-changing healthcare systems in which we work and as a reflective leader we can develop a team reflexivity approach which, according to Dayan and Basarir (2008), is anticipated to have a positive effect on multiple project outcomes and increases the likelihood of produce success, in this situation quality service healthcare provision. However, in order to facilitate this reflexive team, the leader needs to be aware that everyone in the team has something to contribute (Jonasson et al 2014) and take to heart the feelings, thoughts and behaviours of others in the team (Göker and Bozkuş 2017). It is through this shared experience that team members can help each other to integrate new meanings, gain understanding of their competence and effects another person's thinking (Jonasson et al 2014).

This team approach to learning is a deliberate way of 'reflexive thinking' as suggested by Göker and Bozkuş (2017). Whilst promoting learning and performance in the workplace through reflection and reflexivity is critical for the team at a group level it also plays an important role for the individual (Boud et al 2006; Kolb 1984; Schon 1983; West 1996). The reflective leader can help form and maintain the groups where team reflexivity can be effective by facilitating the members of the team to utilise their unique expertise and integrate the differentiated expertise of other members. It is through a facilitative leadership approach that Hirt et al (2004) argue is associated with team reflexivity. However, the leader needs to be clear about what they are trying to achieve, demonstrate authority and power in order to empower the team and give high-quality interpersonal treatment during the process (Dayan and Basarir 2008) whilst preventing hierarchical patterns from dominating (Jonasson et al 2014; Carlsson et al 2014).

These teams should adopt group strategies, objectives and processes to respond to environmental changes through the use of the transactive memory system (group approach) (Dayan and Basarir 2008). It is only when we reflect on our practice based on our theoretical knowledge, consider the impact our leadership has on others in the team and implement insights gained from meeting to improve our leadership performance can this process be called a professional learning community (Göker and Bozkuş 2017).

This is reflexivity from a community perspective with commitment and learning needs to be supported by the community culture (Wendel et al 2018). This community is created by the leader who can serve as a coach and mentor providing positive reinforcement to the team members (Castelli 2016) through the provision of a safe environment for self-expression and feedback that is supportive and positive (Göker and Bozkuş 2017), and which respects diversity and cultural customs and habits (Castelli 2016).

Team reflexivity also forms an integral part in the process of decision making and leadership. The difference between this, and many of the leadership approaches noted in the first part of the book, is the emphasis on a team/collaborative approach. West (2002) argues that although reflexivity is the property of individual team members, aggregated reflexivity can contribute to team reflexivity whilst Matsuo (2016) argues that the key situational factor that enhances reflection and reflexivity in the team is the leader. Dayan and Basarir (2008) also argue that team reflexivity is significantly related to transactive memory system, goal clarity, team empowerment and interactional justice and produces success if the environment conditions are turbulent.

A reflective leader also needs goal clarity which leads the team to a point where members are able to set clear goals after open-minded discussions of diverse views. This results in interactions among team members becoming more effective which in turn leads to the higher team reflexivity (Dayan and Basarir 2008). Reflective team working becomes goal orientated where everyone is expected to adhere to working methods which have been developed together (Jonasson et al 2014) as discussed in the section below in relation to using our narrative intelligence.

The reflective leader needs to develop ways of reducing barriers within teams, such as different professional backgrounds, levels of practice and teams within and outside of the organisation in which they work. But at the same time being resilient by holding onto our values for practice from whichever background we come from. A reflective leader therefore needs to develop this reflective and reflexive environment where they can establish and articulate personal value systems, show respect to others, draw on strengths and weaknesses of self and others, recognise and meet employees' rights and responsibilities in line with legal and formal requirements and develop workforce relationships rather than focusing on structure and hierarchy (Biddle 2005).

All the approaches to reflection mentioned above, from reflection through different levels to critical/intensive reflection and reflexivity have a place for us as reflective leaders as we move forward in response to the changing, complex and challenging healthcare service delivery in which we work. As Matsuo (2016) argues, reflection and/or reflexivity plays a significant role in enhancing learning both at individual and team levels and transformational or facilitative leadership has a positive impact on team reflection or reflexivity.

Reflective practice

In addition to reflection, levels and reflexivity authors such as Schon (1983, 87), Argyris and Schon (1974) and Redmond (2006) talk about 'reflective practice'. This, according to Göker and Bozkuş (2017), is about professional knowledge and whilst they suggest that scientific knowledge is 'prescribed' by theory, and they argue that professional knowledge is 'informed' by theory. They argue that it is often after actions that realties occur as results, outcomes and consequences, and the realities further affect intentions. Göker and Bozkuş (2017) go on to argue that reflective practice is seen as a transformative process where people can become interconnected, where they can define common objectives and goals.

Göker and Bozkuş (2017) identify that reflective practice aims to create a structure, habit or routine as well as help us to install reflection into our activities that are down to earth and yet come about at the right intervals and with adequate depth to be meaningful. However, they note that it is structured sustaining reflective practice that will transform the probability of learning from our practice into an activity and is the best place that leaders can learn about their theories of practice and learn from experience. Last (2020) postulates that reflective practice presents an opportunity to learn from what went as well as what might be improved in order to identify our learning needs. Reflective practice should be contextualised in work and not be considered separately from the cultural milieu together with the setting and purposes of the organisation (Göker and Bozkuş 2017). Ghaye and Lillyman (2010) discuss the concept of reflective practice further in healthcare through several of their principles of reflection for healthcare professionals.

In order to facilitate reflective practice, the leader needs to bring about informal and regular meetings to allow reflective practice whilst providing a safe environment for people to take time for reflective thinking. Just being aware does not always create learning. There is a need to act on the conception that knowledge is planted in our experience and being able to understand the significance of that knowledge fosters our practice. This, according to Göker and Bozkuş (2017), can be achieved through reflective thinking and reflective practice.

Göker and Bozkuş (2017) also argue that the success of reflective practice depends on learning for everyone in the team but that it required us as reflective leaders doing immersed learning. The relationship between experience and reflection is important and to learn from experience requires reflection and it is more than technical and rational knowledge in complex areas of practice (Sullivan and Weissner, 2010). According to Rosenberg (2010), reflective practice serves to identify implicit questions where our choices and decisions are driven by an innate desire to be happy and it is through reflective practice that cultures strengthen the ability to cultivate happiness.

One of the potential barriers that we may encounter as reflective leaders is the culture and organisational values in which we work. This may be due to more competition between trusts and organisations (Kings Fund 2018) as well as professional barriers within the team. However, as argued earlier, the reflective leader has a role to play in creating reflective learning communities and a workplace that encourages reflective practice, includes a safe environment that promotes trust, values open conversations, is able to connect work to the organisation mission, builds confidence of the workforce, respects diverse cultures and challenges beliefs and assumptions.

References

Andersen, T (1987). The reflecting team: Dialogue and meta-dialogue in clinical work. *Family Process*, 26(4), 415–428.

Anderson, H (6 October 2022). Govt warned NHS may be forced to 'completely revisit' investment plans. *HSJ*. www.hsj.co.uk/finance-and-efficiency/govt-warned-nhs-may-be-forced-to-completely-revisit-investment-plans/7033397.article (Accessed 24/01/23).

Argyris, C, Schon, D (1974). *Theory in Practice: Increasing Professional Effectiveness*. San Francisco: Jossey Bass.

Atkins, S, Murphy, K (1994). Reflective practice. *Nursing Standard*, 8(39), 49–56.

Biddle, I (2005). Approaches to management: Style of leadership. *Business*, 13(3), 1–4.

Boud, D, Cressey, P, Docherty, P (2006). *Productive Reflection at Work.* London: Routledge, 3.

Carlsson, G, Hantilsson, U, Nyström, M (2014). Reflective team – a clinical intervention for care improvement. *Reflective Practice International and Multidisciplinary Perspectives*, 15(3). 378–389. 10.1080/14623943.2014. 900008.

Carmeli, A, Gelbard, R, Reiter-Palmon, R (2013). Leadership, creative problem-solving capacity, and creative performance: The importance of knowledge sharing. *Psychology Faculty Publications*, 50. https://digitalcommons.unomaha.edu/psychfacpub/50.

Carter, SM, West, MA (1998). Reflexivity effectiveness and mental health in BBC-TV production teams. *Small Group Research*, 29, 583–601. 10.1177/1 046496498295003 (Accessed 24/01/23).

Castelli, PA (2016). Reflective leadership review: A framework for improving organisational performance. *Journal of Management Development*, 35(2), 217–236. 10.1108/JMD-08-2015-0112.

Cressey, P, Boud, D (2006). The emergence of productive reflection. In Boud, D, Cressey, P, Docherty P (Eds.) *Productive Reflection at Work: Learning for Changing Organisations.* London: Routledge, 11–26.

Cunliffe, AL (2004). On Becoming a critically reflective practitioner. *Journal of Management Education*, 28(4), 407–426.

Cunliffe, A (2009). Reflexivity, learning and reflexive practice. In Armstrong, SJ, Fukami, CV (Eds.) *The SAGE Handbook of Management Learning.* London: SAGE.

Darzi, A (2008). *High Quality Care For All: Next Stage Review Final Report.* London: TSO. https://assets.publishing.service.gov.uk/government/uploads/ system/uploads/attachment_data/file/228836/7432.pdf (Accessed 24/01/23).

Dayan, M, Basarir, A (2008). Antecedents and consequences of team reflexivity in new product development projects. *Journal of Business and Industrial Marketing*, 25(1), 18–29. 10.1108/08858621011009128.

Department of Health (2010). *Equity and Excellence: Liberating the NHS.* London: The Stationery Office. https://assets.publishing.service.gov.uk/ government/uploads/system/uploads/attachment_data/file/213823/dh_ 117794.pdf (Accessed 24/01/23).

Dewey, J (1933). *How We Think: A Restatement of the Relation of Reflective Thinking to the Educative Process.* Boston, MA: D.C. Heath.

Dixon, M, Lee, S, Ghaye, T (2016). Strengths-based reflective practices for the management of change: Applications from sport and positive psychology. *Journal of Change Management*, 16(2), 142–157. 10.1080/14697017.2015. 112584.

Ekebergh, M (2001). *Tillägnandet av vårdvetenskaplig kunskap – reflexionens betydelse för lärandet. [The Acquisition of Caring Science in Nursing and Nursing Education – The Importance of Reflection for Learning].* Doctoral thesis. Vasa: Institutionen för Vårdvetenskap, Åbo Akademi.

Flannagan, J (1954). The Critical Incident Technique. *Psychological Bulletin*, 51, 327–358.

Francis, R (2013). *Report of the Mid Staffordshire NHS Foundation Trust. Public Inquiry*. London. The Stationary Office.

Fredrickson, B (2009). *Positivity: Ground Breaking Research Reveals How to Embrace the Hidden Strength of Positive Emotions, Overcome Negativity, and Thrive*. New York, NY: Crown.

Fredrickson, BL (1998). What good are positive emotions. *Review of General Psychology*, 2, 300–319. Retrieved from 10.1037/1089-2680.2.3.300.

Fredrickson, BL (2001). The role of positive emotions in positive psychology: The broaden-and-build theory of positive emotions. *American Psychologist*, 56, 218–226. Retrieved from 10.1037/0003-066X.56.3.218.

Fredrickson, BL (2003). The value of positive emotions. *American Scientist*, 91, 330–335.

Fredrickson, BL (2004). The broaden-and-build theory of positive emotions. *Philosophical Transactions at the Royal Society of London series B – Biological Sciences*, 359, 1367–1377. 10.1098/rstb.2004.1512.

Fredrickson, BL, Losada, MF (2008). Positive affect and the complex dynamics of human flourishing. *American Psychology 2005 October*, 60(7), 678–686. 10.1037/0003-066X.60.7.678. https://www.ncbi.nlm.nih.gov/pmc/articles/PMC3126111/pdf/nihms305179.pdf.

Ghaye, T (2011). *Teaching and Learning Through Reflective Practice: A Practical Guide for Positive Action*. Abingdon: Routledge.

Ghaye, T, Lilleyman, S (2006). *Learning Journals and Critical Incidents, Reflective Practice for Health Care Professionals* (2nd Edition). Quay Books.

Ghaye, T, Lillyman, S (2008). *The Reflective Mentor*. Quay Books.

Ghaye, T, Lillyman, S (2010). *Reflection: Principles and Practice for Health Care Professionals* (2nd ed). Dinton: Mark Allen Publisher.

Gibbs, G (1988). *Learning by Doing: A Guide to Teaching and Learning Methods*. Oxford: Oxford Further Education Unit.

Göker, S, Bozkuş, K (2017). Reflective Leadership: Learning to manage and lead human organisations. In Alvinius, A (Ed.) *Contemporary Leadership Challenges*. Intech Open. available at https://cdn.intechopen.com/pdfs/52166.pdf. 10.5772/64968 (accessed 20/10/22).

Göker, SD (2012). Reflective leadership in EFL. *Theory and Practice Language Studies*, 2(7), 1355–1362. 10.4304/tpls.2.7.1355-1362.

Goodman, J (1984). Reflection and teacher education, a case study and theoretical; analysis Interchange 15, 9-26 cited in Jasper M (2003) Beginning reflective practice. Foundations in nursing and healthcare. Cengage Learning Emea.

Goodman, RM, Speers, MA, McLeroy, K, et al. (1998). Identifying and defining the dimensions of community capacity to provide a basis for measurement. *Health Education Behaviour*, 25(3), 258–278.

Gray, DE (2007). Facilitating management learning developing critical reflection through reflective tools. *Management Learning*, 38(5), 495–517. 10.11 77/1350507607083204.

Herold, DM, Fedor, DB, Caldwell, S, et al (2008). The effects of transformational and change leadership on employees' commitment to a change: A multilevel study. *Journal of Applied Psychology*, 93(2), 346–357. 10.1037/ 0021-9010.93.2.346.

Hirt, MJK et al (2004). Capacity building the self-reflective leader. *Public Manager*, 86(1), 12–16.

Horton-Deutsch, S (2013). Thinking it through: The path to effective leadership. *American Nurse Today*, 8(8). https://www.myamericannurse.com/ thinking-it-through-the-path-to-reflective-leadership/ (Accessed 10/04/23).

Isen, AM, Labroo, AA (2003). Some ways in which positive affect facilitates decision making and judgment. In Schneider, SL, Shanteau, J (Eds.) *Emerging perspectives on judgment and decision research*. Cambridge University Press. 365–393. 10.1017/CBO9780511609978.013.

Johns, C (2004). *Becoming a Reflective Practitioner* (2nd ed). London: Blackwell Science.

Jonasson, LL, Carlsson, G, Rydström, I (2014). Prerequisites for sustainable care improvement using the reflective team as a work model. *International Journal of Qualitative Studies on Health and Well-Being*, 9, 23934. 10.3402/ qhw.v9.23934.

Jonasson, LL, Nyström, M, Rydström, I (2017). Reflective team in caring for people living with dementia: A base for care improvement. *Reflective Practice*, 18(3), 397–409. 10.1080/14623943.2017.1294534.

Kember, D, Leung, DY, Jones, A et al (2000). Development of a questionnaire to measure the level of reflective thinking. *Assess Evaluation in High Education*, 25, 381–395.

Kember, D, McKay, J, Sinclair, K et al (2008). A four-category scheme for coding and assessing the level of reflection in written work. *Assessment & Evaluation in Higher Education*, 33(4), 369–379.

Kemmis, S (1985). Action research and politics of reflection. In Boud, D, Keough, R, Walker, D (Eds.) *Reflection Turning Experience into Learning*. London: Kogan Page.

Keogh, B (2013). *Review into the Quality of Care and Treatment Provided by 14 Hospital Trusts in England: Overview Report*. London: NHS England. https://www.nhs.uk/NHSEngland/bruce-keogh-review/Documents/ outcomes/keogh-review-final-report.pdf (accessed 29/01/23).

Kings Fund (2018). Leadership in today's NHS. Delivering the impossible. Available at: https://www.kingsfund.org.uk/sites/default/files/2018-07/ Leadership_in_todays_NHS.pdf (Accessed 29/10/22).

Kolb, DA (1984). *Experiential Learning: Experience as the Source of Learning and Development*. Englewood Cliffs, NJ: Prentice-Hall.

Last, R (2020). Patient Unmet Needs (PUNS) and Professional Education Needs (PENS): Using reflective practice to identify your learning needs. *Practice Nurse Journal*, 50(8), 30–35.

Looman, MD (2003). Reflective leadership strategic planning from heart and soul. *Consulting Psychology Journal Practice and Research*, 5(4), 215–221.

Mann, K, Gordon, J, MacLeod, A (2009). Reflection and reflective practice in health professions education: A systematic review. *Advanced Health Science Education Theory Practice*, 14, 595–621.

Matsuo, M (2016). Reflective leadership and team learning: An exploratory study. *Journal of Workplace Learning*, 28(5), 307–321. 10.1108/JWL-12-2 015-0089 (accessed (29/10/22).

Mezirow, J (1991). *Transformative Dimensions of Adult Learning*. San Francisco, CA: Jossey-Bass.

Moon, JA (1999). *Reflection in Learning and Professional Development*. London: Kogan Page.

Moon, JA (2004). *A Handbook of Reflective and Experiential Learning: Theory and Practice*. London: Routledge.

Ngugen, QD, Fernandez, N, Karsenti, T et al (2014). What is reflection? A conceptual analysis of major definitions and a proposal of a five-component model. *Medical Education*, 48, 1176–1189. 10.1111/medu.12583.

NHS England (2016). *Leading Change, Adding Value*. https://www.england.nhs.uk/wp-content/uploads/2016/05/nursing-framework.pdf (Accessed 24/01/23).

NHS Improvement (2016). *Implementing the Forward View: Supporting Providers to Deliver*. https://assets.publishing.service.gov.uk/government/uploads/system/uploads/attachment_data/file/499663/Provider_roadmap_11feb.pdf (Accessed 24/01/23).

Oeij, PRA, Gaspersz, JBR, van Vuuren, T, Dhondt, S (2017). Leadership in innovation projects: an illustration of the reflective practitioner and the relation to organizational learning. *Journal of Innovation and Entrepreneurship*, 6, 2. 10.1186/s13731-017-0062-3.

Peltier, JW, Hay, A, Drago, W (2005). The reflective learning continuum: Reflecting on reflection. *Journal of Marketing Education*, 27(3), 250–263. 10.1177/0273475305279657.

Redmond, B (2006). *Reflection in Action: Developing Reflective Practice in Health and Social Services* (2nd ed.). Aldershot: Ashgate.

Reynolds, M (1998). Reflection and critical reflection in management learning. *Management Learning*, 29(2), 183–200.

Reynolds, M (1999). Critical reflection and management education: Rehabilitating less hierarchical approaches. *Journal of Management Education*, 23, 537–553. 10.1177/105256299902300506.

Rolfe, G, Freshwater, D, Jasper, M (2001). *Critical Reflection in Nursing and the Helping Professions: A User's Guide*. Basingstoke: Palgrave Macmillan, 34–36.

Rosenberg, LR (2010). Transforming leadership: Reflective practice and the enhancement of happiness. *Reflective Practice*, 11(1), 9–18.

Rosenberg, M (1990). Reflexivity and emotions. *Social Psychology Quarterly*, 53(1), 3–12.

Rucinski, DA, Bauch, PA (2006). Reflective ethical and moral constructs in educational leadership preparation: Effects on graduates' practice. *Journal of Educational Administration*, 44(5), 487–508.

Sandars, J (2009). The use of reflection in medical education: AMEE Guide no. 44. *Medical Teacher*, 31, 685–695.

Schön, DA (1983). *The Reflective Practitioner: How Professionals Think in Action*. New York, NY: Basic Books.

Schön, DA (1987). *Educating the Reflective Practitioner: Toward a New Design for Teaching and Learning*. USA: Jossey-Bass inc.

Schwahn, CJ, Spady, WG (1998). *Total Leaders: Applying the Best Future-Focused Change Strategies to Education*. Arlington: VA American Association of School Administers.

Stroebel, CK, McDaniel, RR, Crabtree, BF, Miller, WL, Nutting, PA, Stange, KC (2005). How complexity science can inform a reflective process for improvement in primary care practices. *The Joint Commission Journal on Quality and Patient Safety*, 31(8), 438–446. 10.1016/s1553-7250(05)31057-9.

Sullivan, LG, Weissner, CA (2010). Learning to be reflective leaders: A case study from the NCCHC Hispanic leadership fellows program. In Wallin, DL (Ed.) *Special Issue: Leadership in an Era of Change. New Directions for Community Colleges, No. 149*. San Francisco: Jossey-Bass, 41–50. 10.1002/cc.

Van Manen, M (1995). On the epistemology of reflective practice. *Teachers and Teaching: Theory and Practice*, 1, 33–50.

Wendel, ML, Castle, WGR, Ingram, BF et al (2018). Critical reflexivity of communities on their experience to improve population health. *American Journal of Public Health*, 108(7), 896–901. 10.2105/AJPH.2018.304404.

West, MA (1996). Reflexivity and working group effectiveness: A conceptual integration. In West, MA (Ed.) *Handbook of Group Psychology*. John Wiley and Sons Chichester, 555–579.

West, MA (2002). Sparkling fountains or stagnant ponds: An integrative model of creativity and innovation implementation in work groups. *Applied Psychology An International Review*, 51, 355–387.

White, S, Fook, J, Gardnder, F (2006). Critical reflection: A review of contemporary literature and understandings. In White, S, Fook, J, Gardner, F (Eds.) *Critical Reflection in Health and Social Care*. Maidenhead: Open University Press, 3–20.

Chapter 4
Becoming a reflective leader

Having reviewed the approaches in the previous chapter we can summarise the characteristics of the reflective leader and whilst some are shared with other approaches noted earlier in the book, we have determined that the reflective leader needs to:

- use conscious activity of purposeful personal reflection (Jonasson et al 2014; Castelli 2016) and be wholehearted in the dedication to reflective processes (Sullivan and Weissner 2010)
- demonstrate a holistic view of leadership (Castelli 2016) drawing on different appropriate leadership styles
- seek universal truths, listening to their inner, intuitive voice (Looman 2003), be open minded to alter views (Sullivan and Weissner 2010), be involved in a continuous process of critical self-awareness and development (Göker and Bozkuş 2017), be self-aware, mindful and develop personal wisdom (Castelli 2016)
- be consistent in their behaviour and self-assured when trying out new behaviours (Castelli 2016; Göker and Bozkuş 2017)
- be a role model, relationship builder, show integrity, with open-door policy and display transparency (Castelli 2016)
- be aware and attentive to experience with people in our daily life (Göker and Bozkuş 2017)
- be actively developing future leaders by nurturing others and becoming involved in the moment and interpreting its adaptive importance (Looman 2003)
- empower others (Göker 2012; Castelli 2016)

DOI: 10.4324/9781003324560-4

- be culturally sensitive and self-monitoring, challenging culturally learned assumptions (Castelli 2016; Göker and Bozkuş 2017)
- be a credible communicator by being an attentive and empathetic listener (Castelli 2016; Göker and Bozkuş 2017)
- connect to work organisation mission, build self-esteem and confidence, challenge beliefs and assumptions (Castelli 2016)
- develop respect for staff, drawing on their strengths and weakness, recognise employees' rights and responsibilities along with legal and formal requirements and meet those needs, and realise that the development of workplace relationships is more vital than the emphasis on structure and hierarchy (Biddle 2005)
- manage conflicts, model and adaptive capacity (Göker and Bozkuş 2017)
- accept and actively encourage follower's constructive criticism (Castelli 2016)
- create a collegial and safe environment (Jonasson et al 2014; Castelli 2016)
- offer mutual support through more thorough reflection (Jonasson et al 2014)
- prompt improved thinking skills together with self-understanding making informed and logical decisions whilst working with others (Göker and Bozkuş 2017)
- be co-creators of change, accepting that any individual or circumstance cannot move out of their individual pace or competency and also be able to communicate those feelings to other people (Göker and Bozkuş 2017; Horton-Deutsch 2013)
- be resilient, flexible and adaptable (Timmins 2015) and active in the search for truth (Sullivan and Weissner 2010)
- be able to vision process or a bigger process of cultural or organisational change (Göker and Bozkuş 2017)
- promote reflective learning and facilitative team reflexivity (Carmeli et al 2013; Hirt et al 2004; Schippers et al 2008)
- lead one's life with presence and personal mastery, to be aware and attentive to our experience with people in our daily life and regard leadership from the standpoint of human experience (Göker and Bozkuş 2017)
- mediate external development frameworks, include creative mediation, addressing internal and external requirements in light of particular context (Warwick and Swaffield 2006; Kings Fund 2018).

Reflective leadership using your:

Emotional intelligence

Emotional intelligence was first introduced by Mayer and Salovey in 1997 into academia and outside of academia by Goleman (1995), and, more recently into healthcare (Freshman and Rubino 2002). Heckemann et al (2015) noted that it is becoming increasingly popular within nursing leadership and is a self-development construct aimed at enhancing the management, of feelings and interpersonal relationships. Goleman (1998) also notes that the most effective leaders score high in emotional intelligence and Lerner and Li (2014) notes that emotion is an important factor in decision making and as Horton-Deutsch and Sherwood (2008) argue reflection has been suggested to foster emotional competent nurse leadership.

Emotional intelligence involves self-awareness, mindfulness, wisdom and good judgement (Castelli 2016) which fits with Göker and Bozkuş (2017, p. 32) definition of the reflective leader who should 'engage in a continuous process of maintained critical self-awareness and development', and Castelli (2016) who states that it should involve an understanding of values and trust in internal thought processes.

Emotional intelligence is not unique to the reflective leader and is used within the resonant leadership, authentic leadership and servant leadership as discussed earlier.

The first quality noted by Castelli (2016) for emotional intelligence is that of self-awareness. As noted previously, this is a requirement for the reflective leader and is achieved through self-reflection and restless self-examination with a policy of openness (Göker 2012). It is reliant on others and a need to be open and receptive to other people's opinions (Göker and Bozkuş 2017). Göker and Bozkuş (2017) go onto suggest that it involves being aware of our own natural talents, exploring personal strengths and having a thorough knowledge of our own gifts and talents can help us identify any weaknesses and align goals and jobs with personal talents. This self-knowledge includes self-awareness, self-understanding and self-management and is an element that if not present will make it difficult for leaders to understand their strengths and weaknesses (Göker and Bozkuş 2017). They go on to suggest that as reflective leaders we need to observe ourselves to learn, continually test and gain better knowledge of self and to be conscious of other people. As Sullivan and Weissner (2010) also highlight, leaders need to continually clarify personal values and allow time for self-care using reflection as a means of authentication.

This self-awareness can help to develop personal wisdom which, with reflection, is often associated with good judgement (Castelli 2016). Castelli (2016) also suggests that the two should occur simultaneously leading to self-insight and self-examination with the capacity to perceive events from multiple perspectives.

This wisdom and self-knowledge are crucial to building a team which is a fundamental requirement for the effective reflective leader as noted previously. However, practical knowledge is also required in order to motivate others into understanding themselves better and improve themselves (Schön 1983).

A reflective framework can help us explore, analyse and foster our emotional intelligence skills which in turn can assist with strategic workforce planning according to Heckemann et al (2015). A reflective leader should develop empowerment through the management of emotion with skills including self-awareness, the capacity to establish purpose and direction, and motivating and inspiring teams (Warriner 2009; Castelli 2016). Castelli (2016) also suggests that this is due to its reliance on self-awareness, mindfulness, wisdom and good judgement which are viewed as more intrinsic or intuitive leadership characteristics and can, as noted by Göker (2012), develop a readiness for change before undertaking larger complex processes.

The reflective leader therefore is reliant on internal thought process as opposed to the external characteristics such as knowledge, experience and intelligence (Castelli 2016) and involves Socratic dialogue in questioning, examining self and searching for inner truth (Sullivan and Weissner 2010). This is discussed further in the section on narrative intelligence.

Castelli (2016) also highlights *mindfulness* as a necessity for reflection and cites George (2012) where they argue that mindfulness teaches us to pay attention to the present moment, they also note that when using this we are able to both participate and observe each moment and at the same time recognise the implications of our actions in the longer term. Quinn (2004) argues that the reflection can increase mindfulness and according to Göker and Bozkuş (2017) requires us to be more fully present in every task in our daily lives whilst developing our emotional intelligence in the process. This can be seen in the reflection-in-action discussed earlier as we are mindful of our practice as it occurs.

Motivating and inspiring teams is also an important process for the reflective leader which involves the ability to plan, have dialogue with others and invite critical feedback without becoming defensive (Rucinski and Bauch 2006). Accepting followers' constructive criticism is important as it can then initiate a positive feedback loop where both parties can respond more openly and not feel personally criticised (Castelli 2016). Göker and Bozkuş (2017) suggest that building professional communities that value learning, acting strategically and sharing leadership and engaging external environments matter to learning and should be one that fosters system learning through evaluation of polices, programmes and resource use, strategic planning endeavours, action research focused on system-wide issues and application of indicators to measure progress towards defined goals. This, according to Sullivan and Weissner (2010), can help with time for self-care where reflection can be used as a means for authentication of personal values as well as empower others and develop a more team approach to leadership to meet the needs of the developing workforce and future leaders.

To achieve the above, the reflective leader needs to be attending to verbal and non-verbal communication when interacting with others, and inquiring and clearing up worries by being an attentive listener (Göker and Bozkuş (2017). This according to Göker and Bozkuş (2017) can be a way of approaching the work of being a leader by leading one's life with presence and personal mastery, it requires learning to be present, to be aware and attentive to personal experience with people in daily life and in it regards leadership from the standpoint of human experience. However, Dixon et al (2016) point out that it can be difficult to think creatively and oppose convention within pressurised and intense conditions.

Emotional intelligence, according to Castelli (2016), can be used through the approach of the reflective leader which they argue offers viable solution towards better understanding of the *cultures and values* of the people and the markets they serve. Closely related to transformational and change management (Castelli 2016). It also helps to describe the task impact on the mission, explain how tasks contribute to goals, relate work to company objectives and acknowledge contributions and views work as purposeful (Castelli 2016). However, the first prerequisite, according to Jonasson et al (2014), is to have a reflective attitude with a willingness to think, problematise and think again by extension, listen in an open and active way that will help incorporate personal values into our practice as reflective leaders.

Appreciative intelligence

Thatchenkery and Metzker (2006) define appreciative intelligence as the ability to see the positive in a situation and then to act purposefully to transform the potential outcomes. They note that this is not just optimism but is a realistic action-orientated process where we develop a course of action to move forward. Using appreciative intelligence can also lead to an appreciative change management process (Ghaye 2011) and help us develop a more strengths-based reflective practice in our management and leadership of change. This model embraces the intention to appreciate and understand our own and others' gifts, talents, limitations, self-worth, identity, role, responsibility and accountability. Change, as Ghaye (2011) notes, is the ability to make the right step rather than about stepping forwards or back.

As noted earlier, reflection should come from a positive experience with more emphasis on the positive than the negative (Fredrickson 2003). However, even when reflecting on the negative we can identify positive aspects of care and build on them. Through the process of building leadership, it should be rooted in knowledge base and analytical skills as well as the ability to integrate theory and practice (Wolfe 2007). As suggested above, this involves shared goals and a permissive interpersonal climate and mutual interpersonal involvement (Jonasson et al 2017). In a rapidly changing system, Rosenberg (2010) argued that a strengths-based approach is more conducive and Hornstrup (2001) cited in Jonasson (2017) notes creative teams can address new tasks and generate new ideas and options in relation to existing tasks.

This appreciative intelligence can be enabled through the use of the way questions are asked within our teams. For example, Orem et al (2007) talked about the power of asking appreciative questions which are carefully phrased to grab the attention to explore more about their personal values and appreciation of themselves, their professional role, their colleagues and the organisation in which they work.

Using Seligman's (2011), PERMA model (Positive emotions, engagement, relationships, meaning and achievement/accomplishment) can help to reflect through a positive lens and help individuals to find their way and flourish resulting in greater happiness, fulfilment and meaning. This in turn can result in people being potentially more receptive to and resilient to change (Dixon et al 2016).

An alternative approach to appreciative intelligence is through the use of storyboarding and narrative intelligence (Lillyman and Bennett 2012). This is discussed further below.

Narrative intelligence

Narrative intelligence is based on our abilities to make sense of our practice and learn from it through the telling of stories and dialogue. Last (2012) noted that the narrative leadership approach involves harnessing the power of storytelling and narrative to improve communication that ultimately can lead to change in practice. Fook (2007) suggests that Schon's approach to tacit or implicit knowledge is embedded in practice which needs to be reflected on to make this explicit in order for improvements to be made which can be achieved through a critical reflective dialogue. Therefore, developing partnerships and working in collaboration with colleagues and teams the reflective leader is able to draw on everyone's expertise in decision making (Biddle 2005; Castelli 2016; Göker and Bozkuş 2017; Jonasson et al 2014; Looman 2003). However, narrative conversations rely on employee commitment and communicating with a strong vision for change through building of supportive relationships with followers (Herold et al 2008) and taking others' experience on board. It is through storytelling and reflective/reflexive conversations that we can develop practice (Gray 2007) where critical reflection incorporates a focus on the questioning of our assumptions and social aspects rather than our individual perspectives. Last (2012) also argues that using narrative leadership skills can help us to create an environment of trust and openness, which inspires and drives better directions for improvement within the service. However, this also involves attention to the analysis of power relations in organisations.

Göker and Bozkuş (2017) note that any discussion and reflection on stories will enrich, change and provide opportunities to install possible changes into practice. Storytelling has been used through the centuries and by many cultures to pass on stories and experiences to each generation and is used regularly in healthcare education (Abrahamson 1998; Hunter 1991; Greenhalgh and Hurtwitz 1999). It is through this process of telling stories that, according to Lottier (1986), we can step back, look at practice and re-arrange it in order to make sense of it. This, as Sternberg (1985) noted, helps with effective function in practice and according to Fornis and Peden-McAlpine (2007) can assist with developing critical thinking. Newman (2003) identified how stories are powerful stimuli and Spouce (2003) used narratives with student nurses to reframe their self-image and develop further understanding of the subject being reviewed. The elements of storytelling and use of narratives are, as Newman (2003) suggested, stories that are processed more fully by the human brain than other stimuli and have a greater impact when the person telling the story recounts their own experience. This then can be embraced by the reflective leader through sharing and learning from each other's past experiences and utilising reflection-on-action.

Peers help clarify our values to match our behaviour (Horton-Deutsch 2013) and Göker and Bozkuş (2017) suggest that critical knowledge includes assumptions, beliefs and values (our ethical knowledge). It is through joint reflection that personal and proven experience can be transformed into shared knowledge (Jonasson et al 2014) which can be shared through reflexive conversations (Gray 2007, Cunliffe 2002). Through this active and purposeful process of exploration and discovery with others, the reflective leader can find unexpected outcomes, and critique where they may have taken-for-granted assumptions before the dialogue. In this instance, it can therefore lead both individuals and team members towards a better understanding. It is by critiquing the presumptions on which beliefs are built that critical reflection encourages learning at a deeper, trans-formative level (Mezirow 1990) as noted previously.

Reflexive conversations may also serve to promote multiple inter-pretations of reality, including critiques of previously uncontested forms of organisational 'truth' (Gray 2007). However, this requires a permissive environment, characterised by openness and positive feelings of co-operation, with generosity and encouragement to open up and talk about thoughts and feelings, this can result in deeper reflection where plans for care can be further developed (Jonasson et al 2014) and where team members can challenge generally accepted norms and ideas (Jonasson et al 2014). Providing a structure that encourages the acquisition of new knowledge can stimulate an interest in it and assist with the reflective and reflexive team learning discussed earlier.

The reflective leader needs to encourage the team to bring their experiences to the surface and further reflect on, and with, them (Jonasson et al 2014). By developing reflective space to focus on values, providing opportunities for meaning-making and space for unfolding of narrative we can move practice forward (Stelter and Law 2010) as noted above. It is the facilitative skills of the reflective leader that can result in positive reflection that can be related to team learning (Matsuo 2016). As Jonasson et al (2014) argue, reflective teams can affect other people's thinking but this requires intertwined listening and thinking and as Pololi et al (2001) suggest group reflection helps decrease feelings of stress and isolation.

Last (2012) reminds us that a narrative can take the form of not just verbal communication but also visual or digital forms. A further approach to storytelling can be through the use of storyboarding as used by Lillyman et al (2010) and Lillyman and Bennett (2012) to develop appreciative intelligence. Developed as a process to encourage learners to use the creative right brain and the critical left brain to formulate ideas in front of a group and then to look at those ideas critically (Lottier 1986).

Therefore, dialogue or discourse through critical reflective conversations, dialogue and/or storytelling is interconnected with critical reflection (Rucinski and Bauch 2006) and can result in meeting the service requirements for the individual receiving care, those giving care and the organisation in which they work. As Last (2012) summarised, the more time we spend in listening, sharing and learning will result in better engagement, improved outcomes and quality of life whilst reducing waste of resources.

Outcomes of being a reflective leader

In summary, if we incorporate our values in relation to the emotional, appreciative and narrative intelligence as a reflective leader we can:

- Create a safe environment that promotes trust within the team and organisation for being open and challenging of our own and others beliefs and assumptions
- develop team learning and new understanding where open conversations and dialogue are valued
- increase the likelihood of product success addressing the challenges of balancing some of the cost-efficient service verses higher quality of care
- develop meaningful solutions and decisions that are embedded in evidence-based practice
- have a goal clarity for self, team and organisation
- Increase our personal and team self-awareness, self-esteem and confidence and improve standards of wellbeing of self and the team
- increase our understanding of obstacles and how to address them with a forward action plan
- Respect each other including diversity, ethnicity, cultures and customs
- Increase our personal and professional development and an interest in learning
- Improve the outcomes for our service users and reduce waste of resources within the service.

However, we must also keep in mind that being a reflective leader does not replace the necessary skills and competence required by effective leaders noted earlier in the book.

References

Abrahamson, C (1998). Storytelling as a pedagogical tool in higher education. *Education*, 118(3), 440. http://www.findarticles.com.

Biddle, I (2005). Approaches to management: Style of leadership. *Business*, 13(3), 1–4.

Carmeli, A, Gelbard, R, Reiter-Palmon, R (2013). Leadership, creative problem-solving capacity, and creative performance: The importance of knowledge sharing. *Psychology Faculty Publications*, 50. https://digitalcommons.unomaha.edu/psychfacpub/50 (Accessed 24/01/23).

Castelli, PA (2016). Reflective leadership review: A framework for improving organisational performance. *Journal of Management Development*, 35(2), 217–236. 10.1108/JMD-08-2015-0112.

Cunliffe, AL (2002). Reflective dialogue practice in management learning. *Management Learning*, 33(1), 35–61.

Dixon, M, Lee, S, Ghaye, T (2016). Strengths-based reflective practices for the management of change: Applications from sport and positive psychology. *Journal of Change Management*, 16(2), 142–157 10.1080/14697017.2015.112584.

Fook, J (2007). Reflective Practice and Critical Reflection. In Lishman, J (Ed.) *Handbook for Practice Learning in Social Work and Social Care, Second Edition: Knowledge and Theory*. Jessica Kingsley, 363–375.

Fornis, S, Peden-McAlpine, C (2007). Evaluation of a reflective learning intervention to improve critical thinking in novice nurses. *Journal of Advanced Nursing*, 57(4), 410–421.

Fredrickson, BL (2003). The value of positive emotions. *American Scientist*, 91, 330–335.

Freshman, BL, Rubino, L. (2002). Emotional intelligence: A core competency for health care administrators. *The Health Care Manager*, 20, 1–9.

George, B (2012). Mindfulness helps you become a better leader. *Harvard Business Review*, 26 October. Available at https://hbr.org/2012/10/mindfulness-helps-you-become-a (Accessed 30/01/23).

Ghaye, T (2011). *Teaching and Learning Through Reflective Practice: A Practical Guide for Positive Action*. Abingdon: Routledge.

Göker, SD (2012). Reflective leadership in EFL. *Theory and Practice Language Studies*, 2(7), 1355–1362. 10.4304/tpls.2.7.1355-1362.

Göker, S, Bozkuş, K (2017). Reflective leadership: Learning to manage and lead human organisations. In Alvinius, A (Ed.) *Contemporary Leadership Challenges*. Intech Open, p. 32. available at https://cdn.intechopen.com/pdfs/52166.pdf. 10.5772/64968 (Accessed 20/10/22).

Goleman, D (1995). *Emotional Intelligence*. New York: Bantam Books.

Goleman, D (1998). *Working with Emotional Intelligence*. New York: Bantam Books.

Gray, DE (2007). Facilitating management learning developing critical reflection through reflective tools. *Management Learning*, 38(5) 495–517. 10.1177/1350507607083204.

Greenhalgh, T, Hurtwitz, B (1999). Narrative based medicine: Why study narrative? *British Medical Journal*, 318, 48–50.

Heckemann, B, Schols, JM, Halfens, RJ (2015). A reflective framework to foster emotionally intelligent leadership in nursing. *Journal of Nursing*

Management, Sep, 23(6), 744–753. 10.1111/jonm.12204. Epub 2014 Jun 19. PMID: 24942539.

Herold, DM, Fedor, DB, Caldwell, S, Liu, Y (2008). The effects of transformational and change leadership on employees' commitment to a change: A multilevel study. *Journal of Applied Psychology*, 93, 346–357. 10.1037/0021-9010.93.2.346.

Hirt, MJK et al (2004). Capacity building the self-reflective leader. *Public Manager*, 86(1), 12–16.

Hornstrup, C (2001). *Development Discussions in Groups-Development Through Dialogue*. Norge: DJØF forlag. Cited in Jonasson LL, Nyström M, Rydström I (2017) Reflective team in caring for people living with dementia: A base for care improvement. *Reflective Practice*. 18(3), 397–409. 10.1080/14623943.2017.1294534.

Horton-Deutsch, S (2013). Thinking it through: The path to reflective leadership. *American Nurse Today*, 8(2). Available at: https://www.myamericannurse.com/thinking-it-through-the-path-to-reflective-leadership/ (Accessed: 10/04/23).

Horton-Deutsch, S, Sherwood, G (2008). Reflection: An educational strategy to develop emotionally-competent nurse leaders. *Journal of Nursing Management*, Nov, 16(8), 946–954. 10.1111/j.1365-2834.2008.00957.x. PMID: 19094107.

Hunter, C (1991). Current Issues in Occupational Health Nursing: A Canadian Perspective. *AAOHN Journal*, 39(7), 313–315. 10.1177/216507999103900702.

Jonasson, LL, Carlsson, G, Rydström, I (2014). Prerequisites for sustainable care improvement using the reflective team as a work model. *International Journal of Qualitative Studies on Health and Well-Being*, 9, 23934. 10.3402/qhw.v9.23934.

Jonasson, LL, Nyström, M, Rydström, I (2017). Reflective team in caring for people living with dementia: A base for care improvement. *Reflective Practice*, 18(3), 397–409. 10.1080/14623943.2017.1294534.

Kings Fund (2018). Leadership in today's NHS. Delivering the impossible. Available at: https://www.kingsfund.org.uk/sites/default/files/2018-07/Leadership_in_todays_NHS.pdf (Accessed 29/10/22).

Last, R (2012). Narrative leadership Using patient stories to shape better services. *Practice Nurse*, 33–37.

Lerner, JS, Li, Y, Valdesolo, P, Kassam, KS (2014). Emotion and decision making. *Annual Review of Psychology*, 66, 799–823. 10.1146/annurev-psych-010213-115043.

Lillyman, S, Bennett, C (2012). Using storyboarding to gain appreciative reflection in the classroom. *Reflective Practice: International and Multidisciplinary Perspectives*, 13(4). 10.1080/14623943.2012.670621.

Lillyman, S, Gutteridge, R, Berridge, P (2010). Using a storyboarding technique in the classroom to address end of life experiences in deeper reflection. *Nurse Education in Practice*, 11(3). 10.1016/j.nepr.2010.08.006.

Looman, MD (2003). Reflective leadership strategic planning from heart and soul. *Consulting Psychology Journal Practice and Research*, 5(4), 215–221.

Lottier, LF (1986). Storyboarding you way to successful training. *Public Personal Management*, 15(4), 421–427.

Matsuo, M (2016). Reflective leadership and team learning: An exploratory study. *Journal of Workplace Learning*, 28(5), 307–321. 10.1108/JWL-12-2 015-0089 (accessed 29/10/22).

Mayer, JD, Salovey, P (1997). What is emotional intelligence? In Salovey, P, Sluyter, DJ (Eds.) *Emotional Development and Emotional Intelligence: Educational Implications*. Basic Books, 3–34.

Mezirow, J (1990). How critical reflection triggers transformative learning. In Mezirow, J (Ed.) *Fostering Reflection in Adulthood: A Guide to Transformative and Emancipatory Learning*. San Francisco CA: Jossey-Bass, 1–20.

Newman, TB (2003). The power of stories over statistics. *British Medical Journal*, 327, 1424–1427. 10.1136/bmj.327.7429.1424.

Orem, SL, Binkert, J, Clancy, AL (2007). *Appreciative Coaching: A Positive Process for Change*. San Francisco: Jossey-Bass.

Pololi, L, Frankel, R, Clay, M et al (2001). One year's experience with a program to facilitate personal and professional development in medical students using reflection groups. *Education for Health*, 14(1), 36–49.

Quinn, RE (2004). *Building the Bridge as You Walk on It: A Guide for Leading Change*. San Francisco: Jossey-Bass.

Rosenberg, LR (2010). Transforming leadership: Reflective practice and the enhancement of happiness. *Reflective Practice*, 11(1), 9–18.

Rucinski, DA, Bauch, PA (2006). Reflective ethical and moral constructs in educational leadership preparation: Effects on graduates' practice. *Journal of Educational Administration*, 44(5), 487–508.

Schippers, MC, Den Hartog, DN, Koopman, PL et al (2008). The role of transformational leadership in enhancing team reflexivity. *Human Relations*, 61(11), 1593–1616.

Schön, DA (1983). *The Reflective Practitioner: How Professionals Think in Action*. New York, NY: Basic Books.

Seligman, M (2011). *Flourish*. New York, NY: Free Press.

Spouse, J (2003). *Professional Learning in Nursing*. Oxford: Blackwell Publishers.

Stelter, R, Law, H (2010). Coaching narrative collaborative practice. *International Coaching Psychology Review*, 5(2), 152–164.

Sternberg, RJ (1985). Implicit theories of intelligence, creativity, and wisdom. *Journal of Personality and Social Psychology*, 49(3), 607–627. 10.1037/0022-3514.49.3.607 (Accessed 24/01/23).

Sullivan, LG, Weissner, CA (2010). Learning to be reflective leaders: A case study from the NCCHC Hispanic leadership fellows program. In Wallin, DL (Ed.)

Special Issue: Leadership in An Era of Change. New Directions for Community Colleges, No. 149. San Francisco: Jossey-Bass, 41–50. 10.1002/cc.

Thatchenkery, T, Metzker, C (2006). *Appreciative Intelligence; Seeing the Mighty Oak as an Acorn.* Oakland CA: Berrett-Koehler Publishers.

The Health Foundation, Strengthening NHS Management and leadership (2022) Available at: https://www.health.org.uk/publications/long-reads/strengthening-nhs-management-and-leadership (Accessed 24/01/23).

Timmins, N (2015). The practice of system leadership. London: The Kings Fund. Available from: https://www.health.org.uk/publications/long-reads/strengthening-nhs-management-and-leadership (Accessed 10/04/23).

Warriner, S (2009). Midwifery and nursing leadership in the ever-changing. *NHS British Journal of Midwifery*, 17(12), 764–771. 10.12968/bjom.2009. 17.12.45544 (Accessed 24/01/23).

Warwick, P, Swaffield, S (2006). Articulating and connecting frameworks of reflective practice and leadership perspectives from 'fast track' trainee teachers. *Reflective Practice: International and Multidisciplinary Perspectives*, 7(2), 247–263.

Wolfe, CJ (2007). The practice of EI coaching in organizations: A hands-on guide to successful outcomes. In Bar-On, R, Maree, K, Elias, M (Eds.) *Educating People to be Emotionally Intelligent.* Portsmouth, NH: Greenwood Publishing Group.

Chapter 5
Positive action as a reflective leader

Positive action as a reflective leader

We have reviewed the application and practicalities of reflective leadership in current healthcare delivery. We have also revisited the different approaches to reflection and how this is linked with and uses emotional, appreciative and narrative intelligence and examples of in- on and before action/practice.

To illustrate this, we will now draw on experiences from a variety of practice settings and from different professional backgrounds using healthcare case scenarios. We note leaders are not just the managers of those who run the organisation but leadership starts with those on the front-line who lead hands on care through to those who are responsible for larger teams and/or organisations. To demonstrate this, we draw on lived experiences from acute, secondary and primary/ community areas of clinical practice.

The scenarios are divided into the areas of being a reflective leader that result in the elevation of positive emotions, develop positivity, build optimism and enhance our resilience.

As noted in an earlier chapter of the book, we will be reviewing the role from a positive, strengths-based approach. These lived experiences identify how we enhance the quality of the care we provide to the people we care for whilst at the same time meeting the current demands of the service in relation to cost-effectiveness.

DOI: 10.4324/9781003324560-5

Leadership and the elevation of positive emotions

Providing care is often very emotional and demanding as healthcare professionals deal with people when they are mainly at their lowest point, often when they are experiencing some physical or mental health issues. It involves not just the people we care for but their families and other carers that are all involved in providing support for their loved ones during these difficult times.

Emotions are often linked to our morale in the workplace and with negative emotions the general morale of the staff and individuals also reduces. Although part of the problem is the workload and type of work being delivered to people it is also linked to stress in the workplace (Hall et al 2016).

It has been widely reported that there is an increase in stress and low morale amongst healthcare staff (Hall et al 2016). This is not unique to the UK but a problem globally in healthcare provision (Chou et al 2014; Portoghese et al 2014). This is often due to 'burnout' amongst staff which is frequently attributed to staff continually working with unmanageable workloads, increasing population with more complex needs and lowering of staffing levels and resources (Hall et al 2016). In addition, Squires et al (2022) noted that the COVID-19 pandemic heightened work-related stress. Hall et al (2016) and Portoghese et al (2014) all link low morale and burnout to patient safety.

WHO (2004) defined the concept of burnout as a 'state of exhaustion' this is not a one off but a continual process where staff are constantly trying to provide a quality service within the stressful environment. Therefore, the reflective leader needs to identify ways of addressing and preventing burnout in the workplace environment.

It is not always possible to find more staff and resources which could address many of these issues so other approaches are required. One approach Portoghese et al (2014) found to help reduce burnout and job strain amongst healthcare staff was to provide them with a sense of control over the situation by promoting autonomy in the workplace.

A further requirement is as Hall et al (2016) reported that we need to develop a workplace that fosters staff wellbeing that helps protect against burnout. This is one where according to the WHO (2010) workers and managers collaborate to produce a continual improvement process that protects and promotes health, safety and wellbeing of all the staff and sustainability of workplace for all who work in the organisation.

In order to elevate the emotions within the workplace, reflective leadership calls for emotional intelligence and sensitivity. This is difficult when the leader is often also part of the team and working in the same workplace setting.

For this, we have identified a situation that could potentially take place in any department/ward/primary/community setting with staff. It is a team meeting that although is normally run monthly due to workload has not been held for the last three months. The staff are tired, burnt-out and angry at the ongoing pressures that they are facing whilst being expected to deliver quality and safe patient care service.

The staff are a mixture of different levels of qualified practitioners and support healthcare workers. Everyone is letting off steam, with good reason, as they feel they are at a point where they cannot provide a good quality service that is safe and effective. Several staff have already left the team thereby creating more of an issue with reduction in staffing levels.

There is the potential that this team meeting can result in a downward spiral of mood if not supported by an empathetic leader. For this situation, the reflective leader will need to use their emotional intelligence, as stated in part two of the book, which has an emphasis on empowerment through the management of emotions (Castelli 2016).

A key part of emotional intelligence is mindfulness. In this situation, the reflective leader needs to pay attention to the present moment as noted by George (2012) by listening to the staff and their concerns and at the same time observing behaviour within the team. It also requires wisdom as noted by Castelli (2016) as this is not the time to introduce new initiatives or dismiss the team's concerns and will necessitate good judgement as to when to intervene in the discussion. Caldwell and Atwijuka (2018) also highlight the importance of acknowledging, validating and truly understanding their colleagues and creating a caring commitment to the staff's wellbeing.

In this situation, we break down the process and review how the reflective leader can use mindfulness and wisdom and how they can acknowledge, validate and demonstrate an understanding in order to elevate the emotions through empowerment, shared goal setting and forward action.

Using mindfulness

At the meeting, the first step is to be mindful of the current situation and as Goleman (1988) states we need to be aware of staff who may be demonstrating what he refers to as 'our two minds'. Whilst staff maybe expressing feelings of anger at the situation there is also commitment to the role they are performing. In this situation, we need to recognise what Goleman refers to as the rational mind verses the emotional mind. He suggests this can lead to a dichotomy between the heart and the head. Here, the staff know that there are no more resources and that you as leader do not have a magic wand but there is also a need to do something to support and evaluate the emotion of the team. It is important not to allow the negative emotions to become more dominant in this situation as feeding the emotional mind can result in ineffectual and irrational thinking.

Using wisdom

Although it is salient to allow staff to 'let off steam', as noted above, there is a need to prevent the situation from escalating and feeding each other's emotional mind. It is also not appropriate to pacify the staff with offers of doing more if it is not within your power. In this environment, we already know there are no staff and recourses available and cannot be called on at that moment to help reduce the workload.

Whilst together in this situation, the leaders can facilitate a narrative dialogue with staff and provide a safe environment for people to voice their concerns.

Acknowledging

Through the active process of listening to the narrative, the leader can give permission for the narrative discussion. We need, as Caldwell and Atwijuka (2018) suggest, a valuing of each other and the contribution that everyone has to play, in this situation by letting people talk and listening to their concerns. By providing space and time you, as leader, are acknowledging their situation and their concerns.

Validating

Through the application of this approach, a leader can validate the team's feelings. By recognising, the frustration and/or anger that is being expressed at the situation. In doing this, the leader demonstrates their value of the individuals within the team as persons with feelings and emotions that affect the care that they provide.

Demonstrating understanding

Having actively listened to the staff, acknowledged their concerns and frustrations and validated those feelings the leader then needs to demonstrate to the team their understanding of the situation but not to offer anything that cannot be achieved or to pacify the staff with platitudes. That would again result in a downward spiral of emotions and feelings of staff leading ultimately to staff sickness and/or reduction in staff retention.

Empowering others

Caldwell and Atwijuka (2018) note the importance of valuing each other and empowering others and affirming them as individuals rather than just part of the team or by the job they do. This can then be interconnected with a team critical reflection (Rucinski and Bauch 2006) which, as noted earlier, can have a positive effect by using the team's unique expertise. However, the leader needs to be clear about what they are trying to achieve, is it just to lift the mood or to provide a way forward for the team? We suggest that working collaboratively towards shared goals and values in this situation will in turn elevate the emotions of the team and ultimately improve wellbeing of the team and safety in healthcare provision.

Goal setting and moving forward

By allowing, listening to and facilitating the dialogue with staff the leader needs to guide it by using appreciative questions that will reframe the outlook. This, according to Ghaye and Lillyman (2008), is not just about seeing things differently but includes choice and should not focus on one issue at the expense of ignoring other aspects. The reflective leader will need to build positive cores and talk about values in relation to understanding the teams and shared values and how they affect their actions. The safe environment of the team meeting needs to provide team members time to explore and try to align their espoused values (what they are saying) with their values in action (what they actually do) and align their individual strengths and collective strengths within the team and the organisation. This approach of using strengths, according to Seligman (2002), can result in work becoming more fulfilling and gratifying.

Strength-based questions in this situation might be: What have you done recently in your role that has enabled you to use your strengths? What have you done recently that you thought had really gone well? What did someone say or do that made you feel that your professional experience was appreciated? In asking people to answer these questions the leader can then explore what these answers tell us about the things that really matter (our values) and the positive actions that we can then put into practice. The leader can then capture the information related to the strengths and appreciation, identifying to the team that there are still positive aspects of practice and values in the work they are doing. The reflective leader can then build on these through reflective conversations or narratives, thereby encouraging team members to believe that there are still positive values, actions and appreciations of their work in the organisation and facilitating strength-based approaches to create an appreciative outlook to their job.

The aim is to bring the team to a position where they can reframe their situation and relook at the problems they are facing from a strength-based positive approach.

Alternative strategy

An alternative strategy in this situation would be to use Marshall Ganz (2011) approach to mobilising the team to achieve purpose when facing conditions of uncertainty. He talks about moving from values through emotion to action. This he suggests can be done through the starting with the story of self (the leader) developing this into the story of 'us' (i.e. the whole team) and making this a story that is relative to the here and now which ends with a call to action that inspires, engages and motivates the team. This involves using the narrative intelligence discussed previously.

The leader, according to Ganz (2011), in this situation tells their story and shares their values through their lived experiences. This can include historical aspects of how we arrived in this situation, what were the influences that bought us here and more importantly where we are going. This is then developed into the story of 'us'. When we share a crisis or situation, he argues, we identify points of intersection where we then link together bringing to the fore the values that then move us as a community rather than individuals. This creates an imperative, a call to action.

Whichever approach is used the aim is to elevate the emotions to a state where the team can then move forward to develop shared goals with a strength-based positive approach. By achieving this, staff become empowered in their role, feel valued within the team and help create an approach that addresses their espoused values and addresses the wellbeing of the individuals within the team.

Leadership that develops positivity

Unlike the situation above where the team are faced with ongoing low morale and negative feelings towards the job, this next situation is when we are faced with a circumstance where we cannot see a positive outcome. As noted in the previous section of the book, we often reflect on the negative aspects of our care and may not be able to see through them. This, according to Schon (1994), can involve reflection-on-action, drawing on past experiences and storytelling to identify how we can change a negative situation into a positive. It very much involves the cycle-based approach which is based on constructive assumptions rather than linear steps (Wright 2009).

Often as healthcare professionals, we find ourselves in crisis situations having to respond with knee-jerk reactions or a firefighting approach to care. We make decisions in the moment when we draw on our experience and expertise to meet the needs. If, however, this did not go to plan, then here is a need to reflect after the event and action plan for future events to prevent a similar outcome.

These incidents are often described in healthcare as 'critical incidents', as first noted by Flanagan and discussed in part two of the book, these are examined following an unexpected death or adverse outcome for a patient.

Whilst we noted earlier that we should attempt to balance our reflections with positive events, there is a need to also reflect on the negative events to prevent repetition and or resulting in lowering morale resulting in the situation noted above. Having said that, we must also be aware not to use the reflection on negative incidents to blame practitioners or as a punishment but to use it as a learning exercise that can then be taken forward in a positive approach to improved care.

For this approach, we are looking at a situation within an acute hospital where an elderly man with vascular dementia has died following a fall after admission. The patient had been admitted from a care home in the night and had been sent from the emergency department to an acute assessment ward and finally onto a medical ward as he had been diagnosed with having had a stroke. There appears to be some confusion within the patient's notes as there is no record of a fall however there is a large bruise and cut on his head. He had been sent for a scan and there was evidence of a bleed in the brain. It was unclear whether the scan was asked for due to the stroke or because the patient had fallen. There had been a verbal handover from the assessment ward that he had fallen but this was not recorded and there was uncertainty whether this had happened in the emergency department, prior to admission or on the assessment ward. Staff from the care home and paramedics who bought him in had no information regarding a fall prior to admission.

As a leader in this situation, whilst there is a need to address the situation and find out where this had occurred, there is a further need to reflect on the incident for future care, record keeping and handover of cases. However, the leader needs to be supportive with a positive attitude towards staff that is transformative, caring, and serving, supporting and encouraging individuals as well as team development (Jonasson et al 2014).

For this, we are using our model of reflective leadership see Figure 5.1.

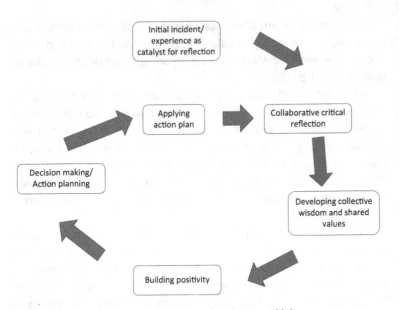

Figure 5.1 Reflective leadership that develops positivity

In this incident, we start the reflection from a point of reflecting on action. The event is past and we are looking towards learning from it and identifying positive ways forward.

Using narrative intelligence, the first part is to review the incident that took place. As stated before, this requires attentive listening by all those involved in the process. It is through the descriptive reflection that occurs here and with narrative intelligence we can start to make sense of the event. As Göker and Bozkuş (2017) tell us, this will enrich, charge and provide us with opportunities to identify any changes that are required into our practice as a team and not in critiquing individuals.

Collaborative critical reflection

Following this stage of description, the team then need to move to collaborative critical reflection. Here, we move from descriptive reflection to critical reflection. As a team, we can question assumptions in practice, review moral as well as technical issues related to the event.

Developing collective wisdom and shared values

The next stage is that of developing collaborative collective wisdom and shared values relating to the incident. At this stage, we are moving towards the process of what Mezirow (1991) referred to as transformational learning. As a team, we can draw on other experiences through other stories where people have experienced similar events or on our professional knowledge in relation to procedures and record keeping. This stage can often result in unexpected outcomes as we explore some of the assumptions that we have about our practice or even learning in relation to procedures such as record keeping and handovers. Through narrative intelligence, we can also at this point help to clarify our values and, as Horton-Deutsch (2013) indicates, then match them to our practice.

Building positivity

We then move onto building positivity. Whilst the incident in this situation has a negative outcome and can result in team and individuals feeling guilty about their care there is also an opportunity to learn and build some positivity into the event.

By using appreciative intelligence, we can draw on what the team and individuals value in this scenario, and how we can then align our espoused values (what we say) with our values in action (what we actually do).

Decision making/action planning

Once people are at this stage, so in the last section, the team can then review the situation from a positive, strength-based approach. From this position, they can make decisions relating to future practice engaging in anticipatory reflection, planning for the next or similar events where they can implement their learning to prevent a similar situation from occurring. At the same time, this provides the learning that will enhance the care and help to put values into practice.

As a leader, we can facilitate this and at the same time be willing to engage in any necessary changes, remaining positive and not causing barriers will assist with the process.

Applying action plan

The final stage will follow the team reflection and is undertaken when the team members come across a similar situation. At this time, they will then have the learning from this event to reflect-in-action and move their practice forward.

Leadership that builds optimism

In this section, we are drawing on Seligman's (2011) PERMA model which was introduced earlier in the book. Here, he identifies five core elements of psychological wellbeing and happiness. He suggests that this can help people reach fulfilment and meaning. His five core elements include: positive emotions, engagement, relationships, meaning and achievement. Rosenberg (2010) also notes that happiness, reflective practice and ethical leadership are all interrelated. Where they suggest that happiness is a dynamic state which enhances personal and organisational change processes.

In the next scenario, we can draw on experiences where we reflect on a situation that had a positive outcome. Whilst we note that these can result in a positive outcome and build optimism for the individual involved they can be used for team reflexivity and building optimism within the team.

By using public narrative as described by Ganz (2011) and appreciative intelligence, the leader can facilitate the reflection that becomes a shared event of learning and moving practice forward.

The scenario here is based in the community where the district nurse is responsible for the care and team providing end-of-life care to a young patient with motor neurone disease receiving end-of-life care at home.

When caring for a person in their home, many different ethical dilemmas and decisions can be encountered that need to be made without the support of other professionals at hand. It will also involve different professionals who may have different values and conflicts in their own approaches to care which is complicated further by being funded by different healthcare bodies, each having different priorities. Any of these can bring our own values and goals into conflict and would need to be managed by the leader of the care.

In this situation, the carer and family were present with the young man during the end-of-life care that he was receiving. As the patient had previously completed an advanced care directive and his wife had lasting power of attorney, there were no conflicts encountered with care provision. He had stated that his preferred pace of care was at home and that there should be no attempt to prolong his life such as resuscitation in the event of an arrest, nasogastric or enteral feeding, he also did not want antibiotics or intravenous fluids when in the final stages of the condition. All staff were aware of the wishes and the wife was also in agreement. Although there were some initial problems getting all the organisations coordinated in providing physical and medical care, due to robust communication and liaison across general practice, community and social care all had gone well and the patient had adequate analgesic and comfort and died with his family by his side and as he had planned.

As this situation was a positive event, it may be overlooked as in a busy work environment we can just move onto the next case. As a reflective leader however we can take these events to reflect and learn from and also build the optimism in the team to continue with their roles. Therefore, using the PERMA approach we can build this optimism in our work.

Positive emotions

Whilst this could be viewed as a sad situation in that a patient has died. The positive elements are that the care provided met the patient's and family's wishes where comfort and dignity was achieved. In this situation, we can end with positive emotions as our values are played out in the scenario. These positive emotions are important for the team and individual and should be shared in the team reflection. As leaders there is a need to feel pride and fulfilment in our role, this is important for wellbeing. It is a situation where we can celebrate our achievements and reflect on the positive outcome.

Engagement

By being involved in the situation either personally or through the sharing of the story in a reflective conversation according to Seligman, we are more likely to experience wellbeing and positivity and optimism in our work. As a leader, facilitating the time out to review, this event provides the opportunity to engage everyone in the event and reflection.

Relationships

Relationships matter and as social beings we can engage in public narrative to share with others. Through sharing and collaborative critical reflection, we are also building our workplace relationships which again are important for our wellbeing.

Meaning

Through the sharing of the incident and reflection, we can then make sense of the event. Putting this into a bigger context, for example, general care for people at end of life in their home environment, we can start to build optimism in the process, resources and outcomes for other patients receiving this care.

Achievement

Acknowledging achievement in the team and individually is an important role for the reflective leader. Using appreciative intelligence in relation to the input of the team into the care given also contributes to optimism and the ability for people and the team to flourish in their work.

Leadership that enhances resilience

Resilience in this situation is not about coping and surviving but about holding onto our personal and professional values and goals through whatever situation we find ourselves in. It is about making sure that we do not lose sight of what our profession is all about, that is the people that it serves are at the heart.

We often have to balance our theoretical, ethical and aesthetic knowledge as noted by Carper (1978) where we have policies and procedures to follow (theoretical knowledge), our own moral beliefs and values (ethical knowledge) and how we behave in the workplace (aesthetic knowledge). Whilst we have the parameters of the policies often in place to protect those using the service this can result in a conflict in our actual beliefs and therefore the act of what we do does not sit comfortably with what we believe. This has been heightened in recent years with the growing culture of litigation and media coverage of the healthcare services. Whilst we have to work within parameters of policy we also need to balance that with the ethical dilemmas that we face in practice when working with other people. Taking a holistic view of our work rather than reviewing conditions and situations in isolation can cause such an issue.

The scenario referred to for this element of enhancing our resilience took place in a large emergency department at an inner-city hospital. Team members were called in as a response to a major incident. Patients had arrived from an incident at a shopping centre and there had been multiple casualties ranging from minor incidents to fatal injuries made up of people from all ages and including several children.

The team had been working at full capacity for several hours in an overcrowded department with distressed families looking for loved ones, police trying to put the incident together and the media attempting to get a story. The team had pulled together. In the debriefing of the event, it became evident that there had been some issues in relation to one of the patients. Whilst all care had been given the staff were informed that one of the patients was in fact the person who had caused the incident by driving their vehicle at people in the car park.

On initial reflection of the incident, the staff expressed how their moral and aesthetic knowledge were now in conflict. As healthcare professionals, they are required to do the best for their patient (aesthetic knowledge), but also they are using resources and time on a patient whose injuries were self-inflicted and at the same time caused harm to others, a conflict to their ethical knowledge (what we value and believe).

Whilst the team had done everything they could for the patient they were now left feeling shocked, confused and frustrated that they had had to spend their time and energy on a person they did not feel was worthy of such attention. The mood was very low and some staff felt guilty for providing the care to this individual.

Referring back to the first approach, the leader needs to facilitate and provide space for people to express their feelings and engage in dialogue, being mindful of and recognising the emotions of the team whilst demonstrating empathy with the situation. These staff were feeling exhausted from the overcrowded department, as noted some felt guilty for using resources and time on an individual they understood had caused the situation, and others were frustrated at the lack of resources and staff available to deal with such a situation.

Whilst the department cannot close for a reflection and other patients need to be seen it is, however, important that the team is given space so as not to allow the situation to become so overpowering and emotional that people leave their shift unsupported and on their own.

This also can be the 'story of now' as noted by Ganz (2011). This, he suggests, will help us to articulate the challenges that the staff face and the choices that they have made in the care that they administered. Also, the meaning of making the right choice even when they feel that they are in conflict with their ethical knowledge. It is through this that Ganz suggests we can draw on those moral sources and find hope and courage to carry on in the role and uphold our values.

Reflective leadership in this situation requires the leader to take responsibility for supporting and guiding staff. Through reflective dialogue and sharing of the stories from the event, the leader can help to unpick the dilemmas and general feelings being expressed in the department. Through appreciative intelligence, they can reframe the situation, recognising the positive elements embedded in the situation and the shared experience of the staff. As noted previously, Thatchenkery and Metzker (2006) argue that using this approach to reframe, appreciate the positive and see how we can inform the future at the same time increases our resilience in practice.

Conclusion

Whichever situation we find ourselves in, we can draw on the approaches included in this section. By using our emotional, appreciative and narrative intelligence, we can build on positive events and bring positivity into events that went well or did not go so well. Our responses and decision making needs to go beyond being impulsive and taking charge, as noted by Dewey (1933) and should 'never' be a checklist but should always consider the complexity of the situation on an individual basis (Warwick and Swaffield 2006).

All practice we encounter provides rich sources of learning even if they are provoked by tension, chaos, struggle, choice, uncertainty, conflict and dilemma. Yet learning from our practice prompted by new situations can result in innovation and creativity and also change our desire to learn more (Wright 2009).

References

Caldwell, C, Atwijuka, S (2018). "I see you!" – The Zulu insight to caring leadership. *The Journal of Values-Based Leadership*, 11(1), Article 13. 10.22543/0733.111.1211. Available at: https://scholar.valpo.edu/jvbl/vol11/iss1/13 (Accessed 24/01/23).

Carper, B (1978). Fundamental patterns of knowing. *Advances in Nursing Science*, 1, 13–23.

Castelli, PA (2016). Reflective leadership review: A framework for improving organisational performance. *Journal of Management Development*, 35(2), 217–236. 10.1108/JMD-08-2015-0112.

Chou, L, Li, C, Hu, SC (2014). Job stress and burnout in hospital employees: Comparisons of different medical professions in a regional hospital in Taiwan. *BMJ Open*, 2014(4), e004185. 10.1136/bmjopen-2013-004185.

Dewey, J (1933). *How We Think: A Restatement of the Relation of Reflective Thinking to the Educative Process*. Boston, MA: D.C. Heath.

Ganz, M (2011). Public narrative, collective action and power. In Odugbemi, S, Lee, T (Eds.) *Accountably Through Public Opinion: From Inertia to Public Action*. Washington DC: The World Bank, 273–289.

George, B (2012). Mindfulness helps you become a better leader. *Harvard Business Review*, 26 October. Available at https://hbr.org/2012/10/mindfulness-helps-you-become-a (Accessed 30/01/23).

Ghaye, T, Lillyman, S (2008). *The Reflective Mentor*. Quay Books.

Göker, S, Bozkuş, K (2017). Reflective Leadership: Learning to manage and lead human organisations. In Alvinius, A (Ed.) *Contemporary Leadership Challenges*. Intech Open. Available at https://cdn.intechopen.com/pdfs/52166.pdf. 10.5772/64968 (Accessed 20/10/22).

Goleman, D (1988). *Working with Emotional Intelligence*. New York: Bantam Books.

Hall, LH, Johnson, J, Wat, I et al (2016). Healthcare staff wellbeing, burnout, and patient safety: A systematic review. *PLoS One*, 11(7), e0159015. 10.1371/journal.pone.0159015 (Accessed 23/01/23).

Horton-Deutsch, S (2013). Thinking through the path to reflective leadership. *American Nurse Today*, 8(2). Available from: https://www.myamericannurse.com/thinking-it-through-the-path-to-reflective-leadership/ Accessed 10/4/23 (Accessed 10/04/23).

Jonasson, LL, Carlsson, G, Rydström, I (2014). Prerequisites for sustainable care improvement using the reflective team as a work model. *International Journal of Qualitative Studies on Health and Well-Being*, 9, 23934. 10.3402/qhw.v9.23934.

Mezirow, J (1991). *Transformative Dimensions of Adult Learning*. San Francisco, CA: Jossey-Bass.

Portoghese, I, Galletta, M, Rosa Coppola, C et al (2014). Burnout and workload among health care workers: The moderating role of job control. *Health and Safety at Work*, 152–157. 10.1016/j.shaw.2014.05.004.

Rosenberg, LR (2010). Transforming leadership: Reflective practice and the enhancement of happiness. *Reflective Practice*, 11(1), 9–18.

Rucinski, DA, Bauch, PA (2006). Reflective ethical and moral constructs in educational leadership preparation: Effects on graduates' practice. *Journal of Educational Administration*, 44(5), 487–508.

Schön, D (1994). Teaching artistry through reflection-in-action. In Tsoukas, H. (Ed.)*New Thinking In Organizational Behaviour*. Oxford: Butterworth-Heinemann, 235–249.

Seligman, M (2011). *Flourish*. New York, NY: Free Press.

Seligman, MEP (2002). *Authentic Happiness: Using the New Positive Psychology to Realize Your Potential for Lasting Fulfillment*. Free Press.

Squires, A et al (2022) How staff burnout and change were escalated by the Covid-19 pandemic. *Nursing Times* [online], 118, 11. Available from: https://www.nursingtimes.net/clinical-archive/wellbeing-for-nurses/how-staff-burnout-and-change-were-escalated-by-the-covid-19-pandemic-31-10-2022/ (Accessed 31/10/22).

Thatchenkery, T, Metzker, C (2006). *Appreciative Intelligence; Seeing the Mighty Oak as an Acorn*. Oakland CA: Berrett-Koehler Publishers. The Health Foundation, Strengthening NHS Management and leadership (2022) Available at: https://www.health.org.uk/publications/long-reads/strengthening-nhs-management-and-leadership (Accessed 24/01/23).

Warwick, P, Swaffield, S (2006). Articulating and connecting frameworks of reflective practice and leadership perspectives from 'fast track' trainee teachers. *Reflective Practice: International and Multidisciplinary Perspectives*, 7(2), 247–263.

World Health Organisation (WHO) (2004). *Organization WH. International Statistical Classification of Diseases and Health Related Problems (The) ICD-10*. World Health Organization.

World Health Organisation (WHO) (2010). WHO healthy workplace framework and model: Background and supporting literature and practices. Available from: https://apps.who.int/iris/handle/10665/113144 (Accessed 24/01/23).

Wright, LL (2009). Leadership in the swamp: Seeking the potentiality of school improvement through principle reflection. *Reflective Practice: International and Multidisciplinary Perspectives*, 10(2), 259–272.

Conclusion

In this book, we have tried to identify the role of the reflective leader within healthcare. We have reviewed the history of leadership within healthcare systems, using the NHS as an exemplar, in order to identify the continual development of the leadership role. Reflective leadership approaches, we argue, can help develop leaders that are able to respond and act in-on and action plan for situations in practice. The reflective leader can at the same time, through using emotional, appreciative and narrative intelligence, facilitate a collaborative and collective approach to leadership that draws on the strengths of those who work within the team and organisation. Consequently, individual, teams and the organisation can develop and balance the ever-changing needs and challenges of healthcare provision or future practice.

Reflective leaders can enable staff to move away from a negative problem-solving approach to care towards feelings of achievements, positivity and optimism in care provision.

Facilitating group and open reflections can be uplifting and enhance learning and help celebrate the care we provide. It can also help to develop leaders of the future that can provide the positive workplace that meets the needs and wellbeing of those who work within it.

It is through this more adaptable approach to leadership that we can think about our practice, not just from a past experience but during events and even before events occur.

The challenge for the reflective leader is to develop the reflective culture within their team, maintaining the forward positive focus towards care provision in a world that continually changes and often includes new and difficult challenges.

Index

Printed in the United States
by Baker & Taylor Publisher Services